SIMPLE PATH

to yoga

SIMPLE PATH

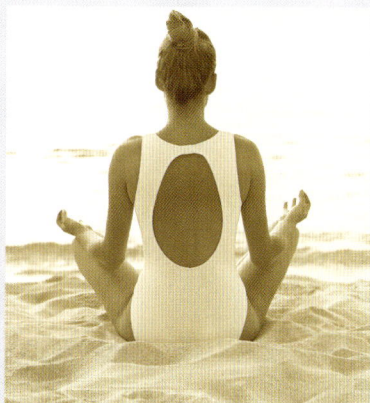

to yoga

Eric Chaline

MQP

First published by MQ Publications Limited
12 The Ivories, 6–8 Northampton Street
London N1 2HY

Text © Eric Chaline 2001
Photographs © Mike Prior 2001
Illustrations © Penny Brown 2001
Design: Justina Leitão and Graham Curd

ISBN: 1 84072 305 X

Printed in China

Contents

introduction

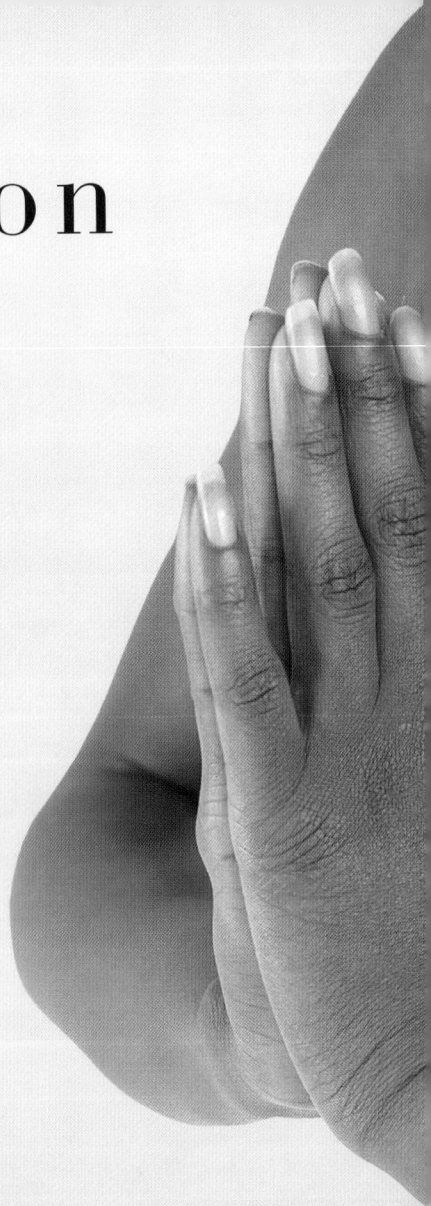

"He who has faith,

who is committed,

and whose senses are

under control,

gains knowledge,

and having obtained it,

he quickly attains

supreme peace."

Bhagavad Gita

a fresh look at yoga

By and large, the books on yoga offer beginners how-to methods, illustrating the principle asanas (postures) of Hatha yoga (yoga of posturing), usually taken from one particular style of yoga, such as Iyengar or Ashtanga yoga (see page 49). Other publications on the subject include learned discussions on the philosophy of yoga, commentaries on the yoga classics, and manuals demonstrating advanced techniques. *Simple Paths to Yoga* aims to bridge the gap between the beginners' manuals, and the more scholarly works. Each of the eight sections introduces a number of yoga techniques, which can be grouped into basic study programs. These include the main asanas (graded easy E, moderate M, and difficult D), pranayama (breathing techniques), bandhas (muscular locks or restraints), and meditation techniques.

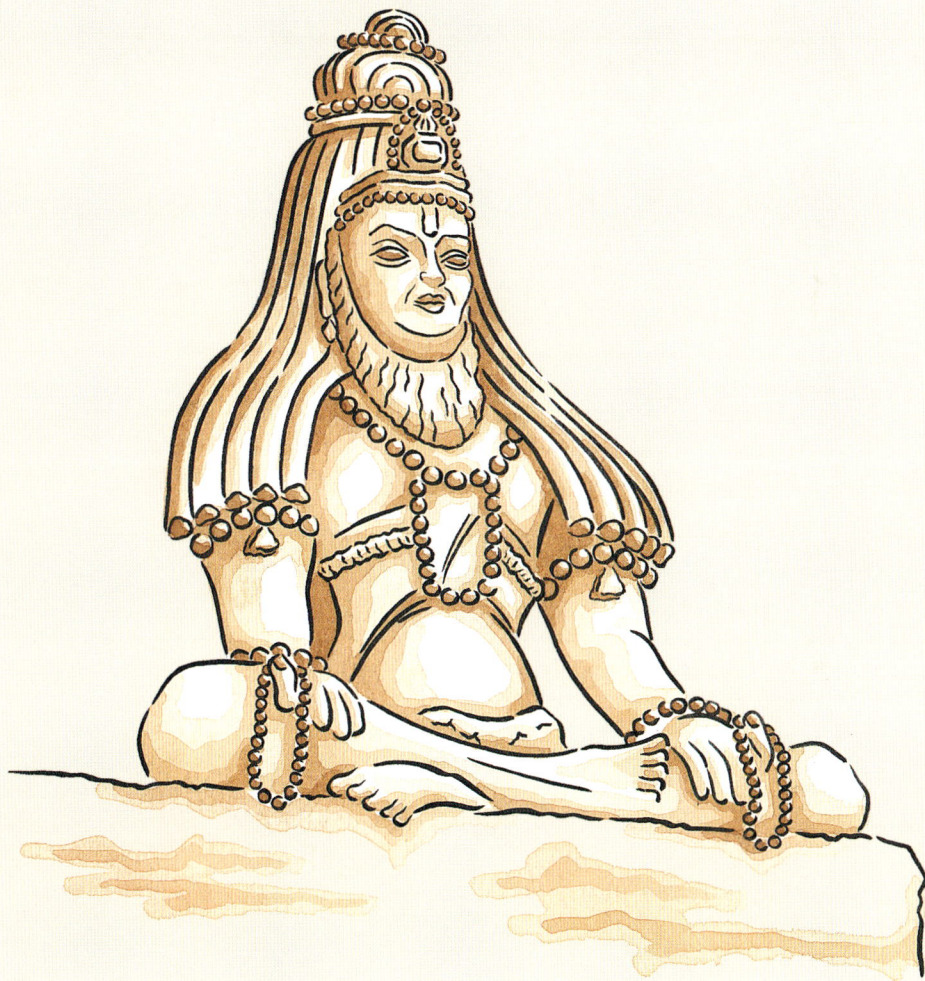

is yoga for me?

We now know that people living the sedentary, high-stress Western lifestyle have to watch what they eat, exercise regularly—in the areas of muscular strength, cardio-vascular (aerobic) fitness, and flexibility—as well as learn techniques to combat stress, if they are to maintain their physical and mental well-being. In short, all aspects of mental and physical fitness have to be addressed to maintain optimum health. The number of exercise options currently on offer is startling. In addition to the traditional team and individual sports and gym, there are exercise classes of every description, and a growing number of non-Western and alternative exercise systems, each claiming to be the fitness equivalent of the "magic bullet" that promises you perfect health, longevity, as well as a toned figure. So how does yoga measure up to the competition? Although it cannot meet everyone's exercise needs, for many yoga will provide training in several vital components of physical well-being:

- Postural alignment
- Flexibility
- Muscular strength and endurance
- Relaxation
- In addition, it will open avenues into a spiritual dimension.

With its emphasis on flexibility, yoga is an ideal complimentary exercise for someone starting out in his or her fitness career or returning to it after an extended break, as well as the more mature exerciser who is entering the latter part of his or her fitness career.

finding the right teacher and class

In India yoga is taught by direct transmission from teacher, or guru, to pupil, or yogi, typically in an ashram (residential community). Each guru will re-interpret the classics in his or her own way, producing an endless number of variations on a common theme. Although there may be differences of emphasis and breathing, the asanas, or physical postures of Hatha yoga remain basically unchanged, regardless of school or style.

As a student in the West you are more likely to attend a weekly class, and it is important to make sure that you find the right teacher and class to suit your personal level and goals. In addition to the style of yoga being taught, each teacher will have his or her own teaching personality. Never take it for granted that he or she is either qualified or a good teacher; make sure by watching a class and asking friends. I have seen people who excelled in their practice of yoga, but were poor teachers, because they could not empathize with students less advanced than themselves. Equally, I have seen teachers, who, although their posturing was not quite as advanced, were truly caring and inspirational.

Ensure that the class is of the right level: do not push yourself beyond your own limits to compete with other pupils or to please the teacher. Yoga, while generally safe, does include particularly challenging stretches, which could lead to injuries, especially for beginners. Always inform your yoga teacher of any injuries you have or problem areas you are experiencing (although a good teacher should ask his or her class, and pay special attention to any problems disclosed).

Yoga was the first of the alternative, non-Western health and fitness systems to come to prominence in the West. During the sixties and seventies, it was taught as a gentle form of stretch and keep-fit, predominantly to middle-aged women. As a result, it was usually adulterated and misunderstood. The growing interest in alternative health and fitness during the eighties and nineties has gone a long way in restoring to yoga its spiritual dimension. It is precisely the readily adaptive quality of yoga that has meant it has evolved through 4,000 years of re-interpretation. Throughout the world today, teachers are constantly developing new yoga styles, adapted to the specific needs of their own culture. For example, a more vigorous form of yoga, "Power" yoga—as physically challenging as aerobics or body-sculpting classes—represents a fresh approach that is in tune with fulfilling the ever growing interest in new Western yoga styles.

practical matters

Hatha yoga is a universal discipline that is not constrained by time, place, or temperature (although heat will facilitate stretching, see page 20).

The ideal place to practice yoga is a quiet, light, and airy location (indoors or out), where you can escape the bustle of the world for the duration of your practice. There is something particularly invigorating about yoga in the open air, with your feet planted on the earth and your head soaring up to the heavens. In cooler weather, practice at the gym or at home.

EQUIPMENT AND CLOTHING

Unlike many other activities, yoga requires little in terms of equipment. A purpose-made yoga mat, which can be bought from any good specialist store, should be long enough to accommodate you stretched out (about

6' x 3'), and can be rolled away easily for storage. A mat is not a necessity and can be substituted with a blanket or rug, but be aware that these may slip or ruck during postures.

Wear clothing that suits the climatic conditions of the location. In cold climates, warm, loose layered clothing is ideal, as it can be removed as the body heats up, and worn again for meditation and breathing exercises. In warmer climates, you may wish to perform the postures semi-clothed, but, whatever the season, do not wear any item of clothing that will constrict the movement of your joints or interfere with digestion or breathing (for example, a tight waistband or an elasticated crop top that constrains the lungs). It is customary to practice yoga in bare feet: it is safer as it lessens the opportunity to slip during poses, and allows for increased sensitivity.

MUSIC AND INCENSE

Some teachers like to use music and incense as part of their practice to create a relaxed atmosphere. Although there is nothing wrong in this, the smell of incense and the sound of music may have the opposite effect from that which was intended—distracting the mind, because the senses become fixated on an unusual experience. You may wish to experiment with your own favorite music, lighting, and room scents but remember that they are merely meant to provide nothing more than a relaxing background to your practice.

TIME

There is no set time of day recommended for the practice of yoga, although several simple common-sense guidelines do suggest themselves. Sufficient time should be left since eating your last meal (at least two hours after a large meal; one hour after a light meal), in order to prevent any discomfort during the asanas that involve twisting and bending the body cavity. Avoid the "down phase" in your daily circadian cycle, when you will not be at your most receptive. The Sun Salutation sequence (pages 288–317) is best practiced while facing the sun in the morning (though not necessarily at sunrise).

HYGIENE

Yoga encompasses a series of hygienic practices—the kriyas—to purify and prepare the body for posturing. These include various forms of internal cleansing (see page 50); only attempt these under the supervision of a qualified teacher. Before starting your practice, you should clear your nasal passages, sinuses, and throat and evacuate your bowels and bladder.

PROGRAMING

Like all forms of exercise, the benefits of yoga are cumulative—the more you practice, the greater the personal benefit. That is not to say, however, that there is no such thing as "too much of a good thing" in yoga (see Caution, page 20). But, unlike running and weight-training, activities to which addictions can be extremely debilitating, the over-enthusiastic yoga practitioner runs few risks.

In terms of frequency of practice, daily practice is the ideal. But whatever time you devote to your practice, make sure that you pursue a balanced program: do not avoid exercises that you find difficult, nor simply favor those that you find easy. You may prefer to perform your pranayama practice at a different time than your posturing: one in the morning, and the other in the evening, for example.

In a cold climate, it is advisable to warm the body up first with gentle stretching and mobility exercises (see the warm-up program on pages 246–57). Guidelines for how long to hold the postures are given with each program on page 246; and several pranayama programs are given on pages 266–73. Three styles of the Surya Namaskar, the Sun Salutation, are illustrated on pages 288–317.

CAUTION

As with all other forms of exercise, due caution should be taken when embarking on a course of yoga study. There are certain conditions, such as high blood pressure (HBP) and problems with the spine and joints, which, although they will be improved by yoga in the long term, could be aggravated by undue straining to attain certain postures at the beginner stage. People with HBP might have problems with the standing asanas (see pages 76–93). Discontinue a posture if you feel light-headed or dizzy. Your breathing should never be labored, and you should never get out of breath. People with spinal problems should be careful when starting the bending and twisting postures (see pages 126–45, and pages 193–205); if you feel any discomfort, discontinue the practice of that asana, and attempt a less taxing pose or warm-up exercise. If you are in a class, follow your own pace—not the teacher's or the other students'—listen to your body and never try to compete with others.

If you are pregnant, consult your medical practitioner before embarking on any of the poses in this book. Equally, if you are a newcomer to yoga practice, and have any doubts about your ability to perform certain exercises, discuss any injury or conditions with a qualified yoga teacher.

"These things are required, first of all: a good place, a suitable time, regulated nourishment and, finally, the purification of the nadis."

Gheranda Samhita

23

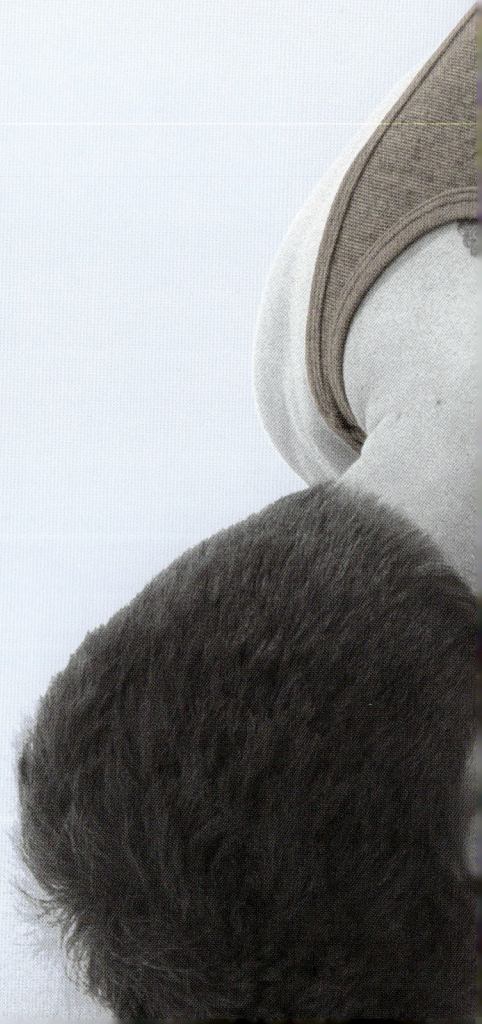

savasana

relax

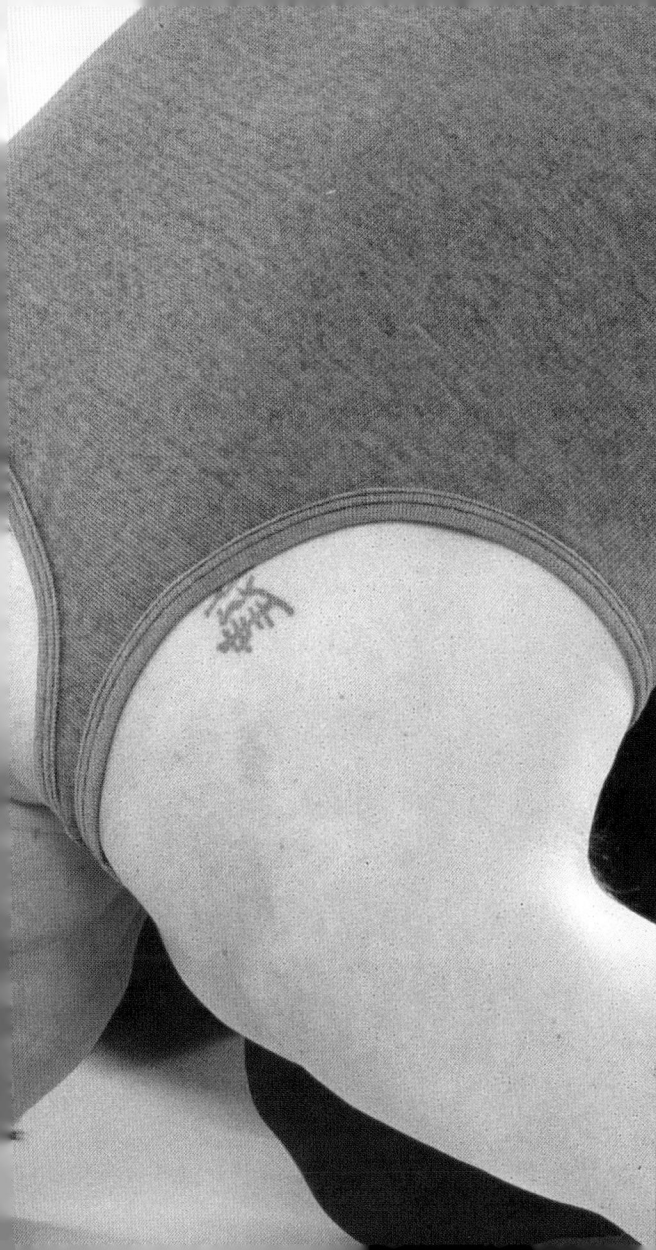

Sava means a corpse.

To lie in Savasana is to

be as still a corpse.

chapter 1

benefits

It may seem strange to some readers to begin a book about exercise with a pose (asana) whose goal is complete physical and mental inactivity. The performance of any sport or exercise, however, will be considerably enhanced if you are mentally and physically relaxed. Focusing the mind will enable you to concentrate all your mental faculties on the task you have set yourself. Reducing physical tension—especially in Hatha yoga with its emphasis on flexibility—will allow your joints to reach their maximum range of motion (see Yoga and Flexibility, pages 146–7), increasing the benefits of the asana, and protecting you from injury.

The immediate benefits of even short periods of relaxation are obvious: a few moments snatched away from the cares and pressures of the world allows the mind and body a chance to rest and revitalize for future challenges. There are many additional benefits, however, about which we may never become fully aware, as the changes are so gradual and subtle. As the only proven remedy for stress that does not involve taking drugs, relaxation will ameliorate any stress-related disorder, including insomnia, depression, lack of energy, digestive and sexual disorders, without the risk of side-effects.

"Lying on the ground like a corpse is called Savasana; it removes fatigue caused by the other asanas and rests the mind."

Hatha Yoga Pradipika

am I tense?

Living hectic but largely sedentary lives, we are only both conscious and completely physically relaxed in the moments just before we fall asleep (you may notice involuntary muscle spasms as the tension held in them is suddenly released the moment at which your body passes from waking to sleep). Although you do not feel the tension in your body, if you are suffering from any kind of stress, it is more than likely that a few of your muscles are in a state of permanent contraction, which, if unchecked, will lead to physical problems.

My study of yoga has been enriched and deepened by an understanding of other bodywork techniques, such as Alexander Therapy, and massage. The greatest contribution to the understanding of muscular tension and relaxation was made by Frederick Alexander; an actor specializing in dramatic monologues, Alexander found that he lost his voice during

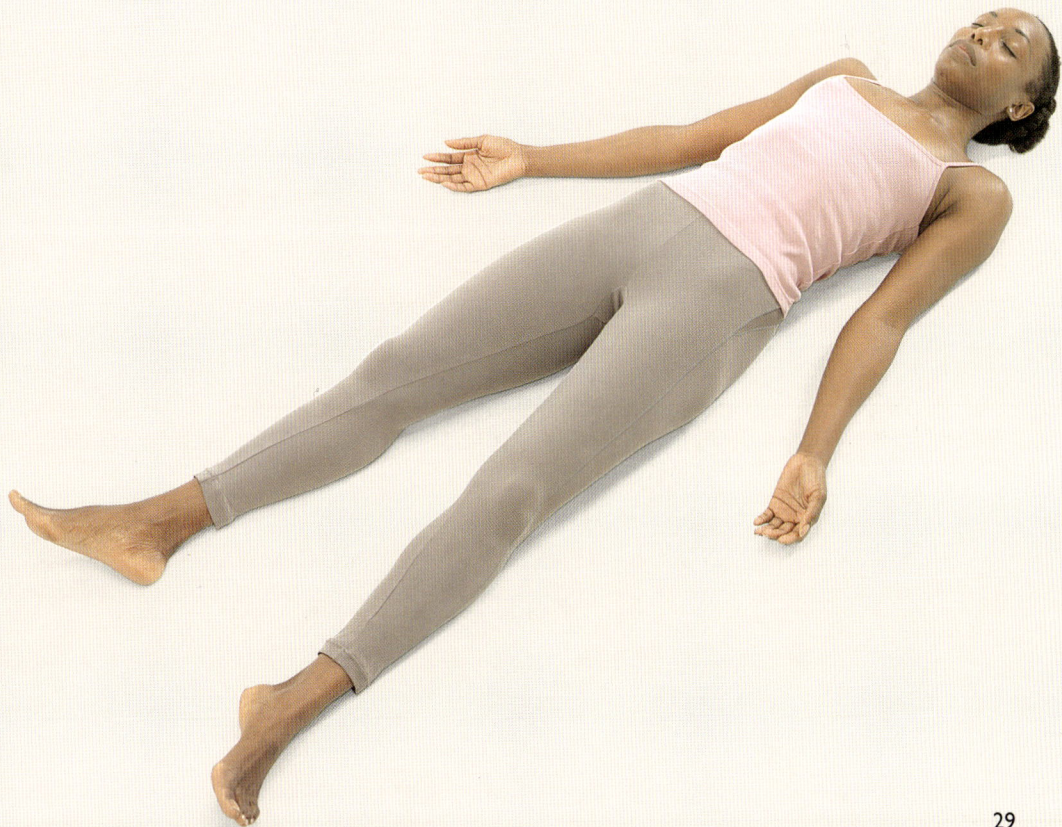

performances. As no doctor could find any obvious cause, he began to observe himself in a mirror. From studying his own reflection, he discovered that both the way he positioned his body, and the pattern of his breathing proved to be the causes of the problem.

The Alexander Technique explains how the "misuse" of our bodies is the source of many of our physical problems. A common example is a person who works at a desk all day working at a PC, sitting with his or her back rounded, head forward and no longer held in balance on top of the spine. In response to the forward position of the head, the muscles of the neck and back will contract permanently to hold the head up. Alexander called this "residual tension." Over a number of years, the body will adapt to the forward position of the head, until it is no longer aware of the tension in the muscles as something abnormal. Unfortunately, the muscles are not designed to be in residual contraction, which, when combined with poor posture, can lead to a range of symptoms, including back and neck pain, and headaches.

The existence of yet another form of deep muscular tension was suggested by Ida Rolf, the creator of a type of massage therapy known as Rolfing. She proposed that when the body is subjected to stress, the fascia—connective tissues within the muscles—lose their elasticity. In a sense, the body acts as a recorder of the emotional stresses we experience. This process is gradual and we are unaware that it is taking place. As in Alexander's theory, the body "adapts," resetting what it feels is "normal."

Whereas both therapies address muscular tension by the direct intervention of a therapist or teacher, the practice of yoga achieves the same ends with its unique combination of relaxation, stretching, muscle toning, and proper posture.

progressive relaxation

In 1938 Edmund Jacobsen devised the "progressive relaxation" method for athletes, consisting of the major muscle groups in the body being tensed and released in turn, enabling you to feel the difference between contracted and relaxed muscles.

A knowledge of basic anatomy will help in your visualization for this exercise, and I have included a basic diagram with the names of the major muscle groups.

MUSCULAR SYSTEM

1. TRAPEZIUS
2. DELTOID
3. PECTORALS
4. BICEPS
5. TRICEPS
6. EXTERNAL OBLIQUE
7. EXTENSORS

8. ANNULAR LIGAMENT
9. GLUTEUS MAXIMUS
10. QUADRICEPS
11. PERONEUS
12. GASTROCNEMIUS
13. SOLEUS

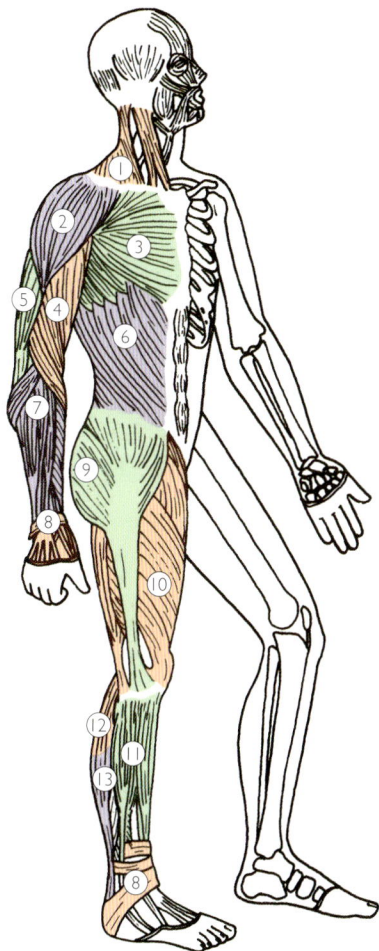

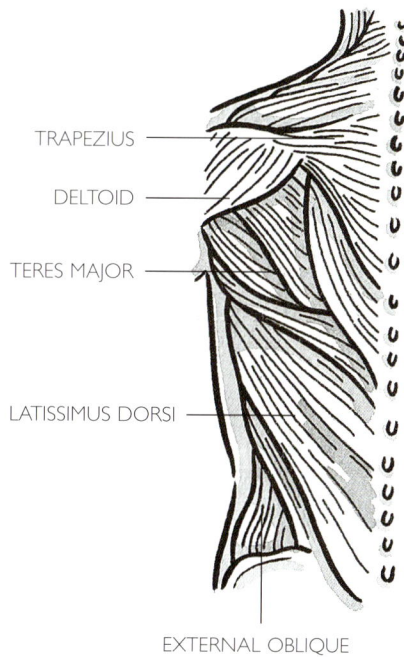

TRAPEZIUS

DELTOID

TERES MAJOR

LATISSIMUS DORSI

EXTERNAL OBLIQUE

PROGRESSIVE RELAXION

- Lying in savasana (see pages 37–43), close your eyes and start to slow and deepen your breathing. Visualize each part of your body in turn, its bones, joints, and muscles, starting at your feet. Breathe in as you tense the muscle, and breathe out as you release it.

Your feet have dozens of small bones, the metatarsals and phalanges. An extremely thick tendon, the Achilles, links your calf muscle to your heel.

- Stretch your feet back and then forward, holding each position for a few seconds before releasing.

Your calves have two muscles: the soleus which lies beneath the gastrocnemius; your thighs have six muscles, three at the front, collectivelty know as the quadriceps, and three at the rear, known as the hamstrings.

- Contract your legs, lifting them an inch off the ground, hold and release.

Your two large buttock muscles are the gluteus maximus.

- Clench these muscles tightly, lifting your buttocks off the ground a little before releasing.

Your back musculature consists of the large V–shaped latissimus and the trapezius muscles.

- Press your whole back into the floor.

- Contract your abdominal muscles, the rectus abdominus and external obliques, hold for 2–3 seconds, and release.

- Tense the pectoralis muscles across your chest, hold and release.

- Contract your arm muscles, the biceps and triceps of your upper arms, and the six muscles of your forearm, lifting your arms about an inch off the ground, hold and release.

- Finally clench your fists tightly, imagining the complex structure of finger muscles and bones closing, hold and release.

RELAXING THE FACE

- Following the same principle as progressive body relaxation on pages 32–35, alternatively contract and release the muscles of your face. As before, without moving your head, tense each area for a few seconds and then release.

- Crinkle your brow. Open your eyes as wide as possible then shut them tight.

- Look far right, and far left, up and down. Smile widely.

- Open your mouth wide, then shut it tightly. With your mouth closed, move your jaw to the right, then to the left

relaxation postures

Relaxation will not only help put your body and mind into neutral, it will also encourage you to be physically receptive to the practice of the asanas, pranayama, and meditation.

The asanas given in this section can be used for two purposes: the relaxation of the body, or the re-alignment and relaxation of the body between physically demanding asanas, such as the bending and inverted postures (see pages 126–45, and pages 156–69). In both cases, you should breathe slowly and evenly, and concentrate your mind on your breath. For example, Balasana, child posture (which is said to be the first asana we ever practice, as it is the position we adopt in our mother's womb) is recommended after Sirshasana; the headstand (pages 164–7), and Pavanmuktasana, the supine knee squeeze posture can be used after Sarvangasana, the shoulder stand and the more demanding bending exercises (see pages 40–1). One exercise from Alexander Therapy, the semi-supine position, will help relax and re-align the body.

37

E

balasana

Child posture

1 Kneel, sitting back on your heels, toes pointing back.

2 Bend forward and place your forehead on the ground. Release all the tension in your torso, and let it sink onto your thighs.

3 Keep your arms by your side, resting easy, palms facing up.

4 Do not jerk out of the posture, but unroll the spine until your back is straight.

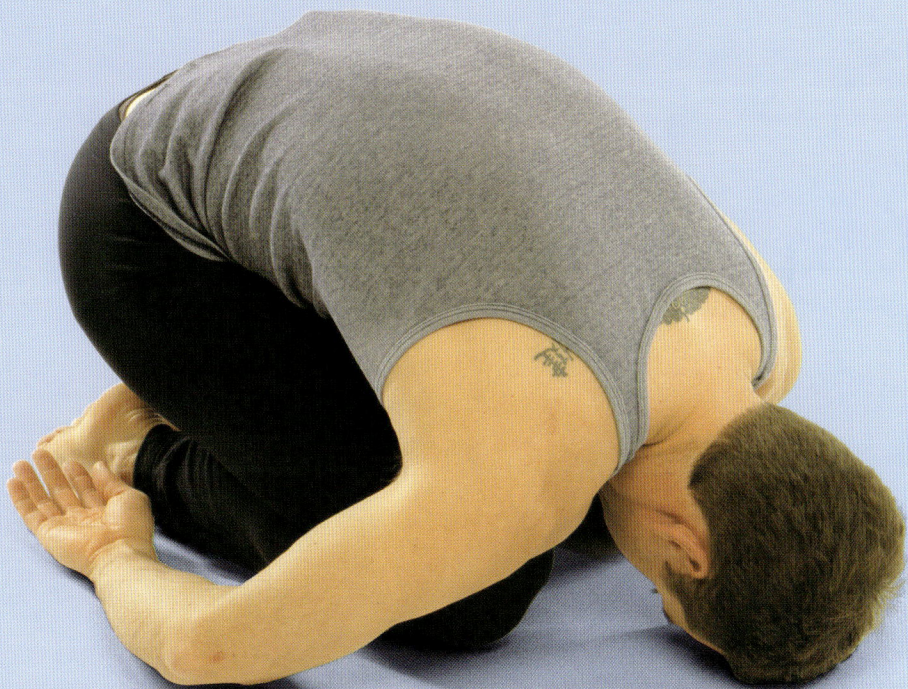

E

pavanmuktasana

Supine knee squeeze posture

1 Lie in Savasana. Draw your legs together.

2 Breathe in as you hug your knees to your chest.

3 In a common variation, breathe out, and raise your forehead (shown here) to your knees as you hug them into your body.

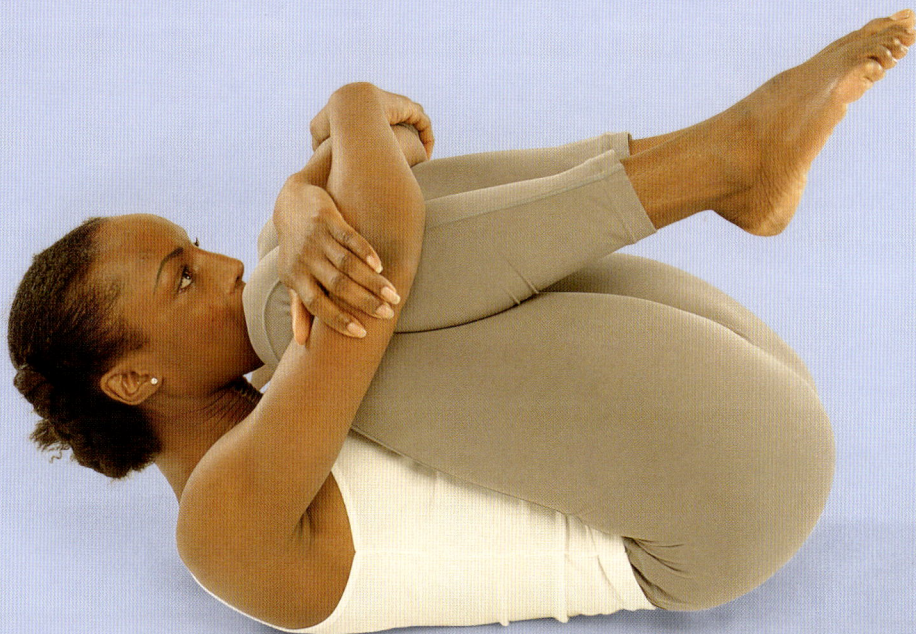

E

Semi-supine position

1 Lie on the floor with your legs outstretched hip-width apart.

2 Bend your legs at the knees and keep your feet flat on the floor. Let your arms rest easy by your side, palms down. Stay in this position for 20 minutes or more, eyes closed, holding the mind steady on your breath.

3 Breathe slowly and evenly through your nose, trying to maintain the same interval for an in- and out-breath.

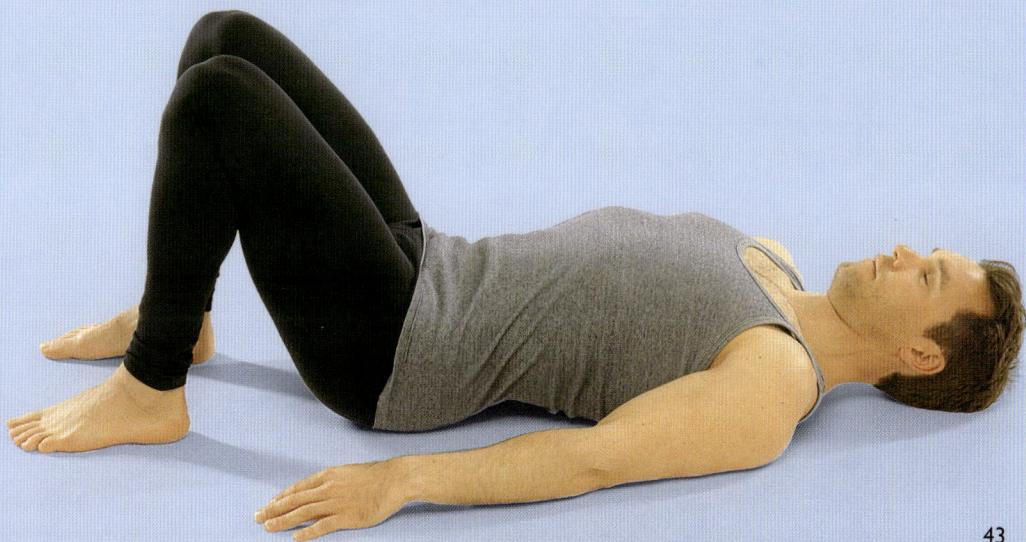

What is yoga?

In its broadest sense, the Sanskrit word yoga, meaning "joining" or "yoking," describes any system of beliefs, religious ritual, or technique, that aims at the transformation of human consciousness to attain Moksha, that is, liberation from the cycle of rebirth, and Samadhi, absorption into Brahman, the ultimate reality. Classical yoga is one of the six darshanas, the schools of Hindu philosophy, whose metaphysical speculations about the nature of reality and existence can be likened to those of the philosophical schools of ancient Greece (see also Hinduism, pages 240–41).

Within yoga itself, there are several paths that share in common the premise to attain the goal of self-realization. They include Jnana yoga, the yoga of wisdom; Raja or Ashtanga yoga, the yoga of meditation; Hatha yoga, the yoga of physical posture; Karma yoga, the yoga of action; and Bhakti yoga, the yoga of religious devotion. In addition, Hinduism recognizes the validity of the three non-Orthodox philosophies: Buddhism, Jainism, and Sikhism, as well as esoteric traditions, such as Tantra yoga (see pages 208–9).

In the West, where yoga has often been taught as a form of fitness training and stretching divorced from its spiritual context, yoga has come to mean the yoga of physical posturing, or Hatha yoga. But this branch of yoga also encompasses a deeply spiritual discipline whose aim is the permanent release of the soul from the earthly plane of existence.

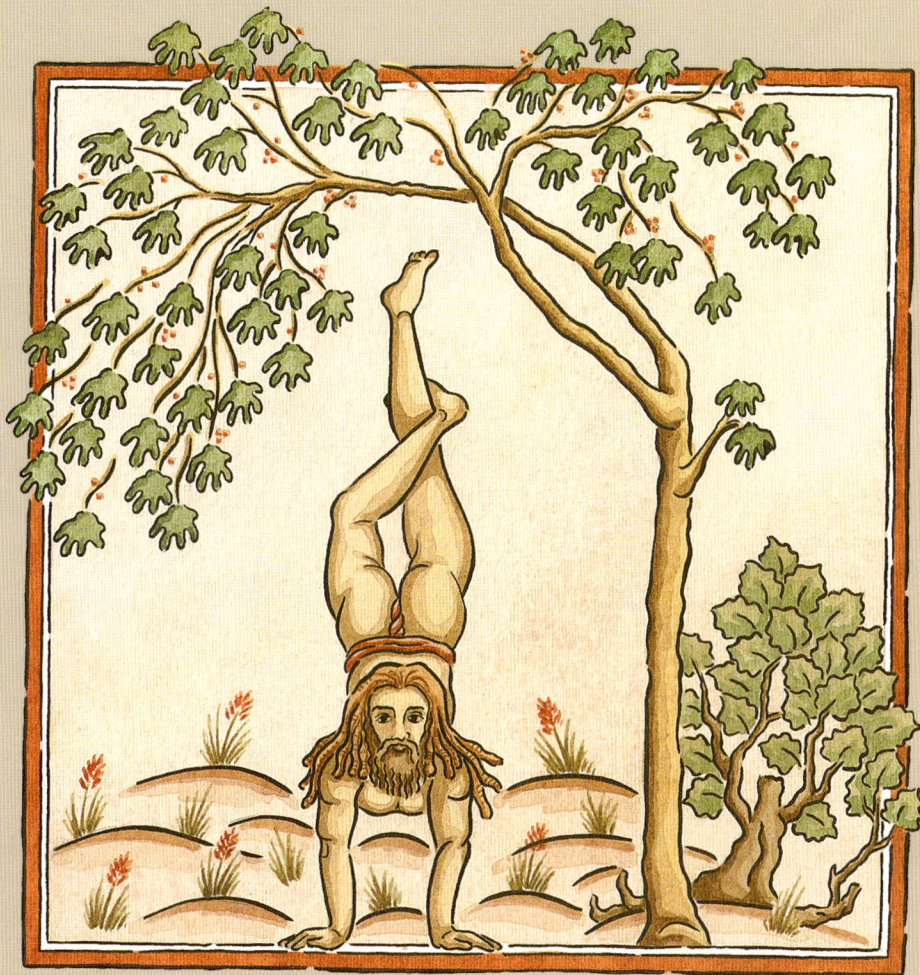

History of yoga

The Indus valley to the northwest of the Indian subcontinent, in the area that is now India and Pakistan, is one of the cradles of world civilization. The world's first cities, Mohenjo-Daro and Harappa, stood here two and a half millennia before the birth of Christ. Although archaeologists know very little about the religious beliefs of these people, they have uncovered figurines seated in postures resembling yoga asanas. After a history of five centuries, whether by alien conquest or natural disaster, the great cities of the Indus went into decline and were abandoned. Their populations were dispersed, leaving the land to the nomadic Aryan peoples of central Asia.

The Aryans brought with them their own gods and customs. They quickly built their own cities and spread to the furthest extremities of the subcontinent. The most ancient Indo-Aryan religious text, the Vedas (eighteenth to fourth century BCE, see page 242) mentions the yoga-like practice of austerities and breathing exercises. However, the first use of the term yoga to describe physical posturing is in a much later set of holy writings, the Upanishads (composed seventh and fifth century BCE, see page 242), in particular, in the Svetasvatara Upanishad, which mentions centering the mind through the control of the body and breath.

Unlike Christianity, Buddhism, or Islam, yoga is not based on the teachings of a single teacher, nor do all yogis share the same philosophical or religious beliefs. Although most believe in a godhead, they may have different conceptions of its nature and role in human affairs. Like Hinduism, yoga is an amalgam of different traditions, which was systematized in various stages. The Maitri Upanishad defines six stages of yoga: breath control, withdrawal of the senses, meditation, concentration, contemplative enquiry and absorption. The two books that have played the greatest role in the definition of Hatha yoga are the Yoga Sutra (yoga aphorisms) of Patanjali and the Hatha Yoga Pradipika (A Lamp for Hatha Yoga) by Svatmarama.

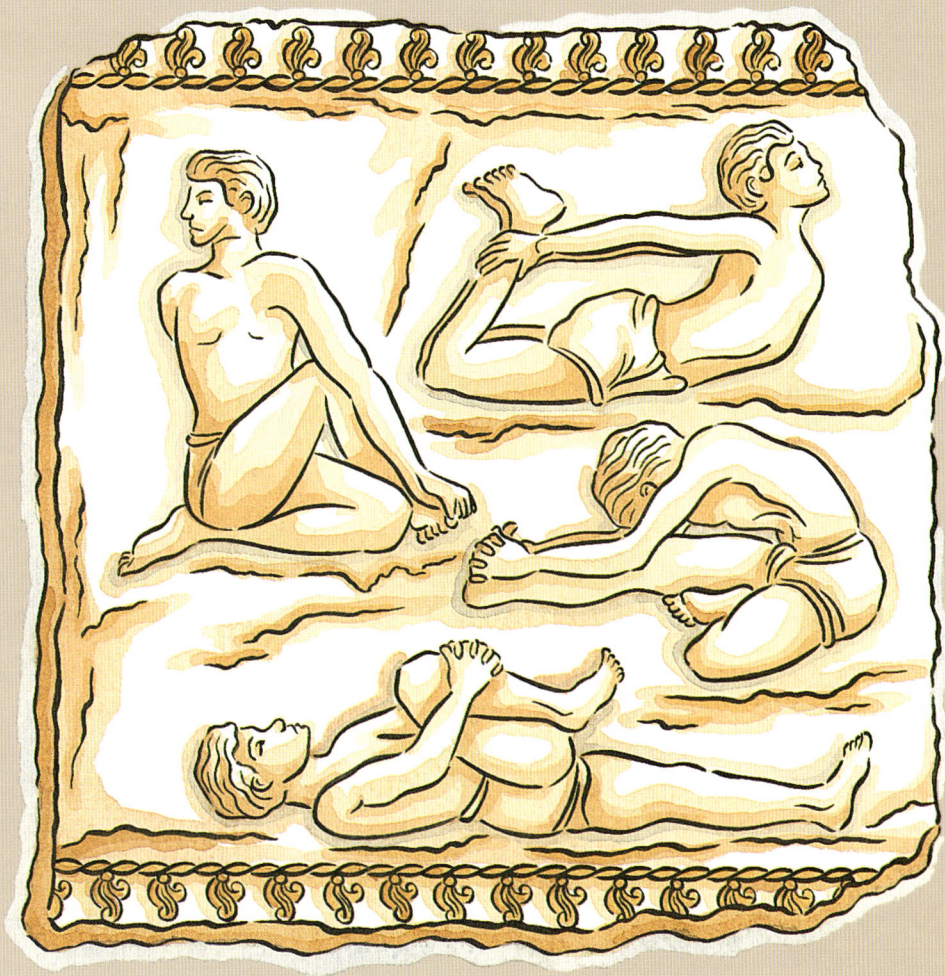

Yoga Sutra of Patanjali

The Yoga Sutra is recognized as the definitive text on the philosophy of classical yoga. The yoga it expounds is sometimes referred to as Raja yoga (royal yoga) or Ashtanga yoga (eight limbed yoga). Almost nothing is known about its author, but it is believed that he lived sometime between the third century BCE and third century CE. The Yoga Sutra consists of 195 short aphorisms divided into four chapters, or padas. The first chapter instructs the yogi on the practices leading to Samadhi (absorption into Brahman); the second chapter defines the eight limbs of Ashtanga yoga.

The last two chapters deal with the subtle states of awareness and advanced techniques of yoga, and Moksha, or liberation. Because of the brevity the verses require interpretation. Important commentaries have been written on the Yoga Sutra in India from the fifth century CE, and these re-interpretations have lead to the creation of new schools of yoga in the modern period. The style of yoga taught in the West as Ashtanga yoga (see page 49) is actually a form of Hatha yoga, which is said by its founder to be based on the principles expounded in the Yoga Sutra.

The Eight Limbs
of Ashtanga Yoga

- YAMA (MORAL OBSERVANCES)
Non-violence, truth, non-stealing, continence, non-coveting

- NIYAMA (SELF-RESTRAINT)
Purity, contentment, austerity, self-study, dedication to god

- ASANA (POSTURES)
Steadiness, health and lightness of limbs; the use of the body to train and discipline the mind

- PRANAYAMA (BREATH CONTROL)
Prepares the mind for concentration

- PRATYAHARA (SENSORY WITHDRAWAL)
Contraction of consciousness from the external world

- DHARANA (CONCENTRATION)
Binding of consciousness to a single point

- DHYANA (MEDITATION)
Overcoming mental fluctuation

- SAMADHI (ABSORPTION)
Absorption of consciousness into Brahman (godhead)

Hatha Yoga Pradipika

The sixteenth century guru, Svatmarama, wrote the Hatha Yoga Pradipika—the principal text on Hatha yoga. It consists of 390 verses divided into four chapters. Although primarily concerned with the physical aspects of yoga, many of its verses also describe the ethical conduct that is expected of a yogi.

The final chapter is devoted to the spiritual discipline of yoga, including sections on pratyahara (withdrawal of the senses), dharana (concentration), dhyana (meditation), and samadhi (absorption), which also feature in the Yoga Sutra.

On the practical side, The Hatha Yoga Pradipika deals with diet, lifestyle, and dwelling place. It describes approximately 40 individual asanas, over 100 pranayama techniques, and over 150 mudras (seals), bandhas (restraints) and internal cleansing practices, as well as the nadis (channels through which prana flows; see pages 56–7) and Kundalini (spiritual energy; see pages 210–13).

The text opens with the asanas, which the author describes as the first "limb" of Hatha yoga. Hatha yoga is sometimes called "six-limbed yoga" (Sadanga yoga), to differentiate it from Patanjali's Ashtanga yoga.

"One should practice
the asanas, which give
the yogi strength, keep him
in good health, and make
his limbs supple."

Hatha Yoga Pradipika

pranayama

breathe

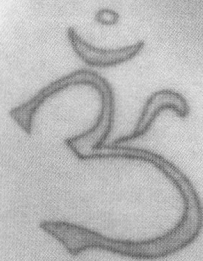

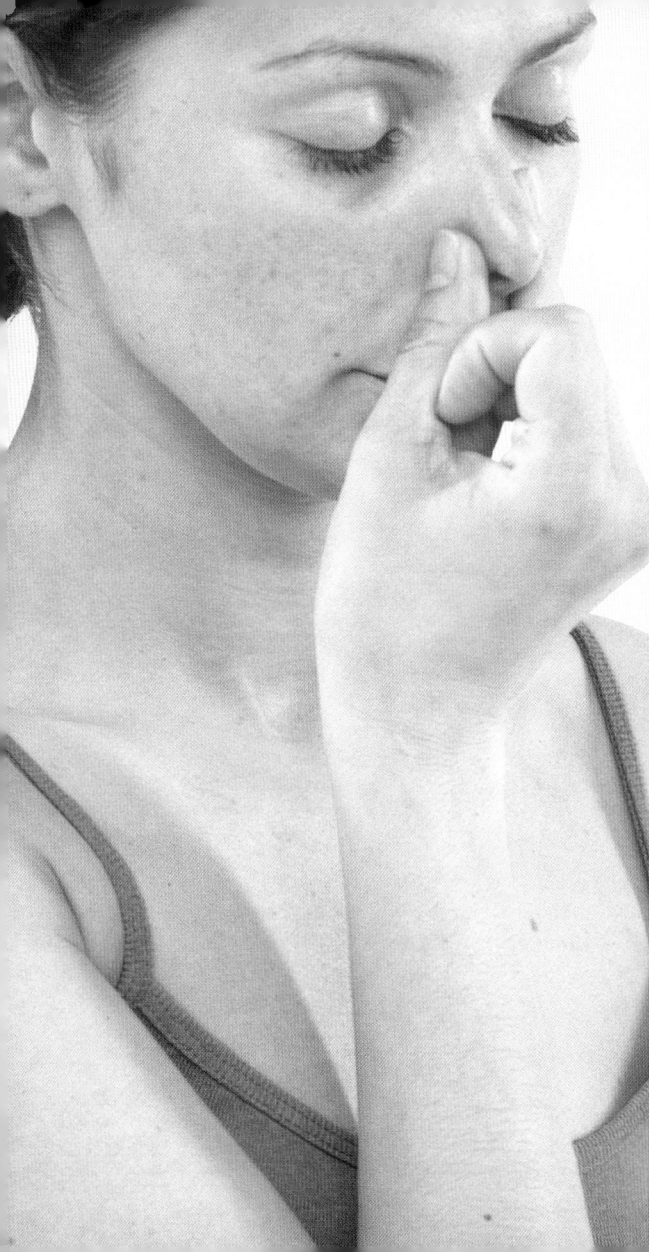

Prana is the life force, vital energy, and breath, and ayama means extension and restraint, thus Pranayama is the control and restraint of the breath.

chapter 2

benefits

Many readers might think that the last thing they need is a lesson in breathing. Breathing is, after all, something all of us have been doing since the day we were born, and as an autonomic (automatic) function of the nervous system, it's not as if we could forget to breathe. We can, however, become bad at breathing. In moments of great stress or emotional disturbance, we are aware of how shallow and quick our breathing becomes, which in extreme cases can reduce the oxygen supply to our brains, and result in anxiety attacks. In such moments, a helpful bystander might advise us to "Breathe, breathe," in order to calm us down.

Panic attacks are, thankfully, extremely rare occurrences; however, the breathing efficiency of many adults who experience low-level stress during work and commuting may be gradually impaired over time, particularly from poor postural habits and residual muscular tension (see page 30).

Regular exposure to air pollutants and irritants, such as carbon monoxide, tobacco smoke, and smog further reduces the efficiency of our lungs.

Although pranayama techniques were not designed to deal with the stresses of modern life, they not only improve the efficiency of our lungs but have also been shown to be remarkably effective as a technique to calm and focus the mind. The regular practice of Pranayama also revitalizes the body and mind by improving the oxygen supply to the organs, tissues, and brain (see Kumbhaka, pages 59–60).

Some yogis believe that our lives are not measured in years, as in the biblical "three score years and ten," but by the number of breaths we take during our own lifetime. Humans are the longest-lived species, they believe, because they take the fewest breaths. In this tradition, the goal of pranayama is to slow the breathing, thereby extending life.

prana

On the purely physiological level, the fourth "limb" of Patanjali's Ashtanga yoga (see page 49), pranayama are techniques that manipulate the breath in order to relax and strengthen the mind and body, in preparation for meditation. In the more esoteric traditions, however, pranayama are used to increase and manipulate the flow of prana, or life force, in the body for both physical and spiritual ends.

It is probably not a coincidence that the Indian concept of prana, which means breath, energy, and the life force, has many similarities with its Chinese counterpart, qi (pronounced chee), as ancient India and China were linked by the Silk Route, which apart from carrying trade goods, was a conduit for religious, social, and scientific ideas. The similarities, however, should not be over-exaggerated, as there are significant differences between the two concepts.

Like qi, prana is the cosmic force that animates the universe. It exists in several forms, notably in the air, from which it is absorbed during breathing, and in the food we eat. Prana flows around the body through channels in the subtle or astral body (see page 171) and can be stored and manipulated to awaken Kundalini, the dormant spirit potential (see pages 210–13).

"As lions and elephants are tamed slowly, so should prana be brought under control according to one's capacity, otherwise it will prove fatal to the practitioner."

Hatha Yoga Pradipika

the stages of the breath

When we breathe, we think of it as a two-stage process in which the in-breaths and out-breaths are of the same duration. In many pranayama techniques, however, a full cycle of the breath is composed of three or four distinct phases, with pauses between in-breaths and out-breaths. The timing of each stage may vary. Some schools of yoga favor a 1-1-1 ratio, while others adopt a 2-8-4 ratio, for in-breath, suspension and out-breath.

PURAKA, OR IN-BREATH

Unless otherwise specified, as in Kapalabhati, the rapid cleansing breath (see page 66), the in-breath should be smooth and even. Do not try to overfill the lungs with air, by bloating the stomach and actively lifting the shoulders. The diaphragm should push down as the ribcage expands outward and the clavicles lift naturally without any conscious raising of the shoulders.

KUMBHAKA I AND II, OR SUSPENSION OF THE BREATH WITH FULL
AND EMPTY LUNGS

Once the lungs are full, many techniques require the breath to be held
for a certain length of time. As a beginner, you will not be expected to
hold your breath for more than a few seconds, but more advanced
practitioners may hold their breath for a minute or more. In this case,
they use Jalandhara bandha, the chin lock (see pages 72–3), to obstruct the
airway and prevent air from escaping or entering the lungs, and also to hold
the prana.

Certain authorities believe that the main physiological benefit of Kumbhaka
is that improves the mixing of new air, rich in oxygen, and the stale residual air
that remains in the lungs after the out-breath, which is much poorer in oxygen
and richer in the waste gas, carbon dioxide.

Kumbhaka II, suspending the breath when the lungs are empty, is obviously a more taxing procedure for the beginner. Do not hold this for more than a few seconds. If you find yourself gasping for breath on the in-breath, you have held your breath too long. With practice, you will be able to hold this stage for longer periods.

RECHAKA, OR OUT-BREATH

The out-breath is considered an important phase of pranayama techniques because this is when carbon dioxide, and other bodily toxins are expelled from the body. Like the in-breath, it should be smooth and unforced. In many techniques the out-breath should be longer than the in-breath. Allow your clavicles to lower, your rib cage to contract, and tense your abdominal muscles but without straining.

pranayama techniques

Pranayama techniques can be used for relaxing, cleansing, or revitalizing the body. For a simple pranayama program, see pages 266–73. Pranayama can be performed after your asana routine, when the body is relaxed and the mind receptive, or at a different time of day, according to your own preference. For time and place etc., follow the same guidelines given in the introduction, pages 15, and 17–18, and for postures suitable for the breathing exercises see the meditation chapter, pages 222–33. Pranayama are deceptively powerful techniques, and people suffering from high and low blood pressure should exercise caution when suspending the breath.

E

Abdominal breathing

I Sit in a comfortable position with your back straight (see pages 78–9 for postures). Dip you head slightly forward, close your eyes. Place your palms on your knees, thumbs touching your forefingers in Jnana mudra (which symbolizes the union of the Atman—the soul, and Brahman godhead), or cupped in your lap.

2 Breathe in slowly and smoothly through your nostrils. Imagine that your lungs are divided into three sections: lower, middle, and upper—that you have to fill in turn. Begin by filling the lower, relaxing your abdominal muscles but without allowing your stomach to bloat, and open the ribcage. Lastly fill the upper chest, allowing your clavicles to rise slightly.

The sequence continues overleaf.

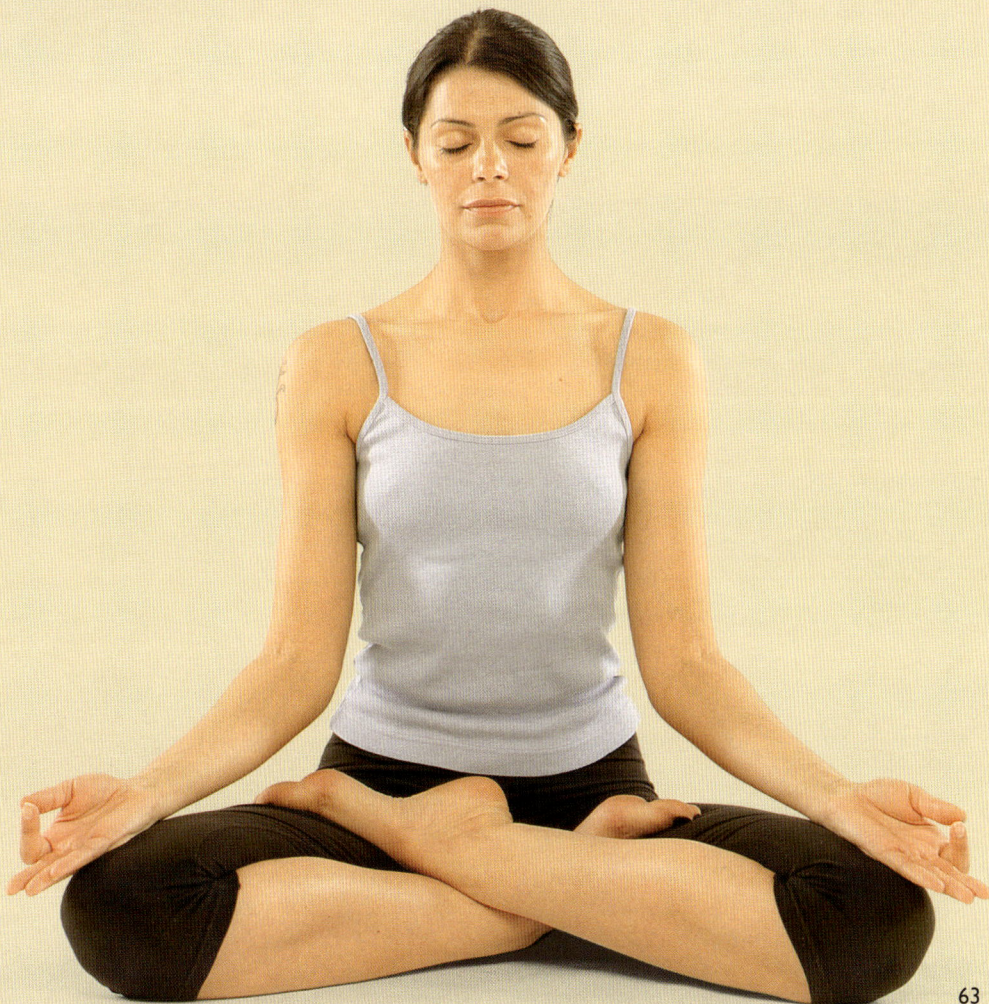

3 Pause for 2–3 seconds before beginning the reverse procedure to empty the lungs fully. As with breathing in, do not exaggerate the movement or strain to expel the air. Keep the pressure smooth and constant and do not over-tense your stomach muscles. Pause again for 2–3 seconds.

4 Try to breathe more deeply, slowly, and smoothly with each breath, until you can breathe in and out for a count of eight. Do not suspend the breath after breathing out for more than a count of three until you have practiced the technique for some time, and feel completely comfortable.

E

Supine abdominal breathing

1 Lie on the ground with your legs hip-width apart. Place one hand on your stomach and the other on your chest. Do not press or put any strength in your hands, as they are merely there to help you monitor your breathing.

2 Follow the instructions for in-breath, pause, and follow with the out-breath, given in Abdominal Breathing on pages 63–4. Feel the rising of your abdomen and rib cage on inhalation and their fall on exhalation. You may wish to experiment with different patterns of breathing, beginning with 1-1-1 (the three phases of the same length), 1-1-2, or 1-2-2.

M

kapalabhati—Cleansing breath

1 In this technique you breathe in and out quickly using your stomach muscles to force the air in and out of your lungs. This exercise is not a pranayama but a krya, or cleansing technique (see page 18), and is usually practiced at the beginning of your session.

2 Sit in a comfortable position, as in Abdominal Breathing. As you breathe out suddenly, contract your stomach muscles, pulling your navel toward your spine.

3 Release the stomach muscles, allowing air to rush into your lungs. Continue for 10–20 breaths, and then rest your lungs with two slow cycles of Abdominal Breathing.

M

ujjayi—Victorious breath

1 Instead of releasing the stomach muscles on the in-breath as in Abdominal Breathing, imagine that your navel and spine are linked by a rope, and that you cannot expand your abdomen.

2 Breathe out fully. Pulling the abdomen in slightly as you breathe in, fill the lungs with air, and feel it lift your chest and back. As you breathe in, the air passing over your palate should make the sound "sa."

3 Hold for a 2–3 seconds, and release the breath, making the sound "ha." Keep the abdomen tight but without straining. Wait 2–3 seconds before taking in the next breath.

D

DIFFICULT TECHNIQUE

anuloma viloma

Alternate nostril breathing

1 In this exercise the thumb and little and ring fingers are used to close the right and left nostrils respectively. In preparation for the first stage of the exercise, close your right nostril with your thumb and breathe out through your left nostril.

2 Breathe in through your left nostril, keeping your right nostril closed (figure 1), filling the three parts of your lungs as in Abdominal Breathing (see pages 62-64).

3 Close the left nostril with your little finger and hold your breath for 2–3 seconds (figure 2).

4 Open the right nostril. Breathe out and breathe in through the right nostril (figure 3).

5 Close both nostrils as before and hold for 2–3 seconds and open the left nostril and breathe out.

This completes a full round of Anuloma Viloma.

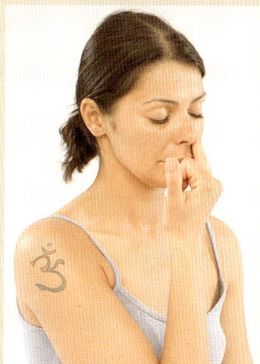

figure 1

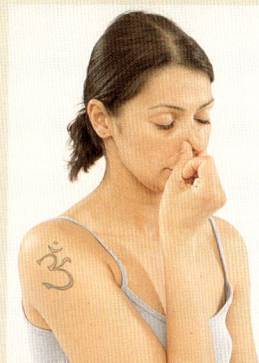

figure 2

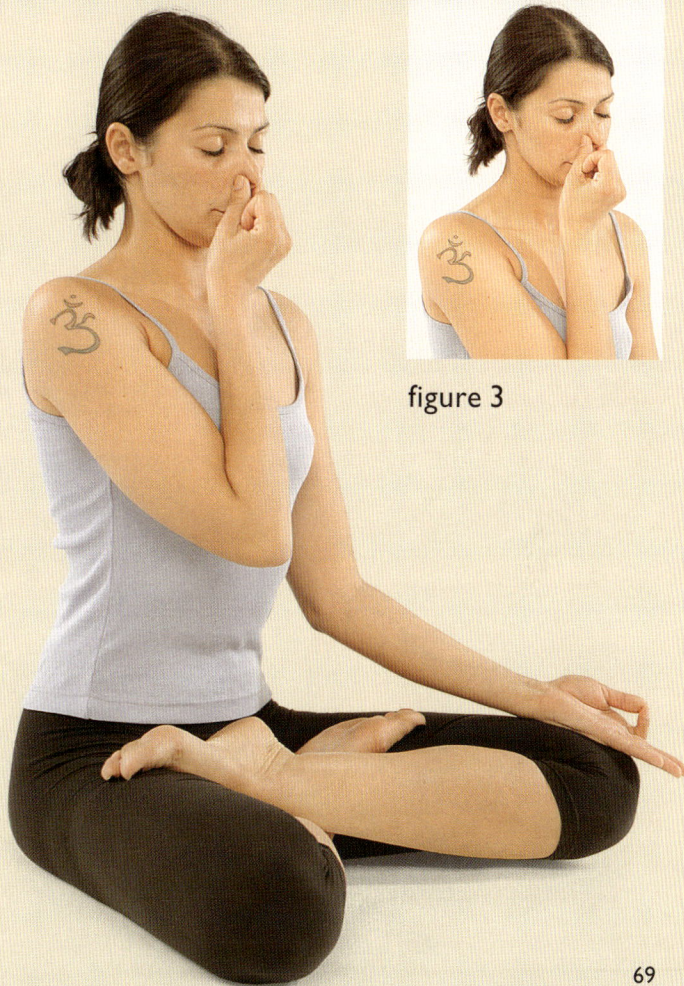

figure 3

bandhas–restraints

In *Light on Yoga*, B.K.S. Iyengar describes the bandhas, or restraints, in the following terms: "When electricity is generated, it is necessary to have transformers, fuses, switches, insulated wires to carry the power to its destination, as without these the electricity would be lethal. When prana is made to flow in the yogi's body by the practice of pranayama it is equally necessary for him to employ bandhas to prevent the dissipation of energy and to carry it to the right quarters without causing damage elsewhere." The three bandhas used during the practice of asanas and pranayama techniques are: Jalandhara, Uddiyana, and Mula.

M

mula bandha—Root restraint

This bandha closes the base of the main energy channel, or nadi, of the astral body (see page 71) that is believed to begin at the base of the spine between the anus and sexual organs, to block the downward flow and dissipation of prana. This restraint is used during asanas and pranayamas, and also during the more esoteric practices of sexual or Tantra yoga (see pages 208–9). Its application is believed to increase sexual vitality.

Adopt a seated position, such as Siddhasana (see pages 222–33), and contract the muscles in the anus and perineum.

M

jalandhara—Chin restraint

In some schools, this is used with the Kumbhaka (suspension) stage of pranayama techniques.

1 Bring the chin down into the notch between your clavicles at the top of the breast bone.

2 With the mouth tightly shut, this effectively seals the windpipe preventing air from entering or departing the lungs.

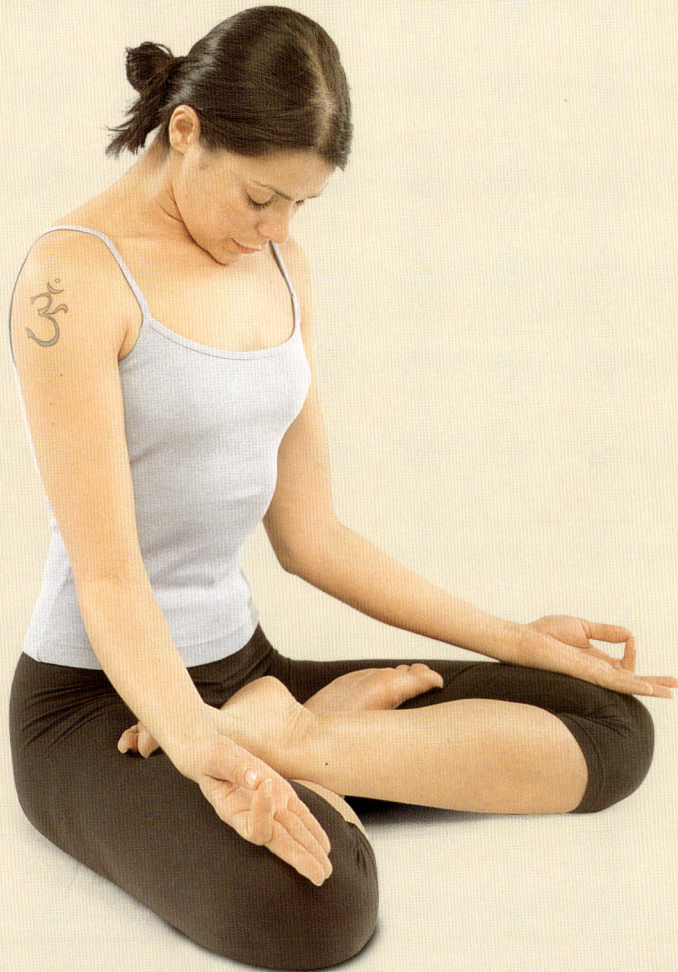

D

DIFFICULT TECHNIQUE

uddiyana bandha

Abdominal restraint

Uddiyana Bandha can be used as an abdominal toning exercise in its own right, and is said to be beneficial to the digestion.

1 Stand feet about hip-width apart. Bend your knees, lean slightly forward, and rest your hands on your upper thighs, fingers spread. Drop your chin to your chest, breathe in and breathe out fully.

2 Hold your breath, pull your stomach in toward the spine, and tighten your abdominal muscles, simultaneously lifting them upward as you press down on your hands that are resting on your thighs.

3 Straighten your body, moving your hands upward from your thighs to your hips. Relax your abdominals and breathe out deeply and slowly.

4 Repeat 5 times to tone the abdominal region.

[Caution: Do not repeat the exercise more than eight times a day.]

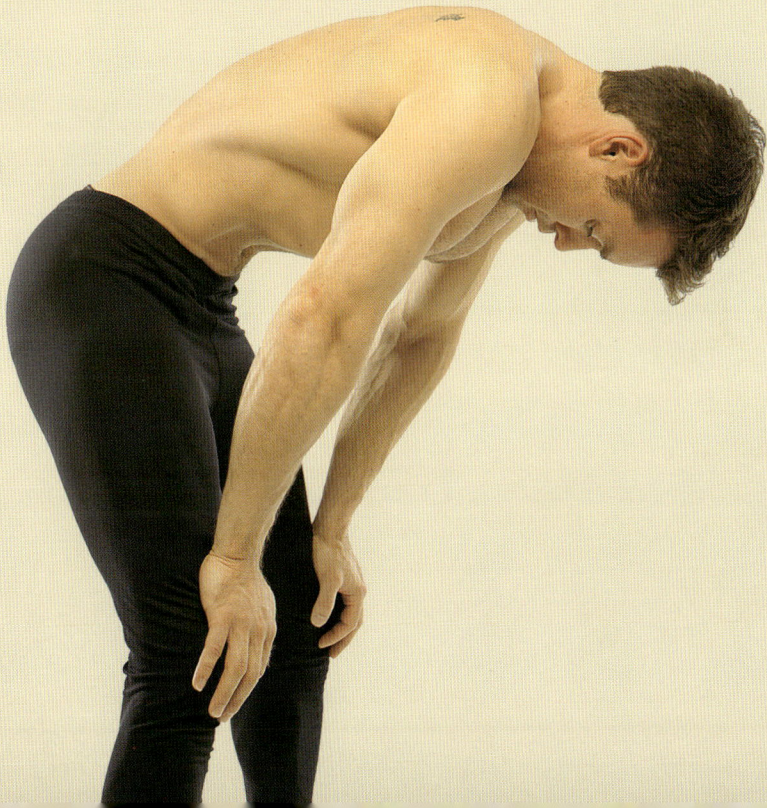

tadasana

stand

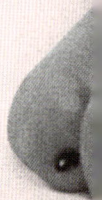

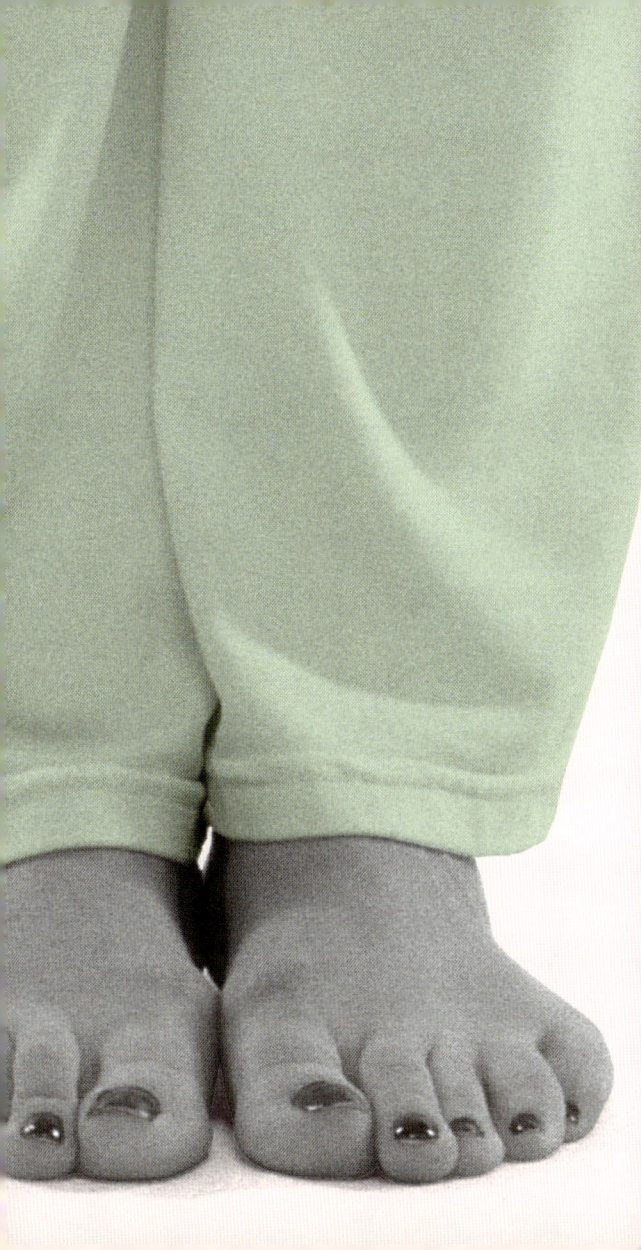

Tada means mountain.
To stand in Tadasana is
to be rooted on the earth
like a mountain.

chapter 3

benefits

"He started with breathing, and now," I hear my reader scoff, "he wants to teach us how to stand!" Naturally, just as we all know how to breathe, we also all know how to stand. But how often have you stopped and consciously thought about the way you stand? As we have seen in the chapter on relaxation, many common ailments are caused by a combination of residual muscular tension and poor posture. A simple way to check your own posture is to stand as you would normally in front of a full-length mirror and observe yourself. Looking at yourself face on, ask yourself:

- *Are my shoulders level, or is one slightly higher than the other?*
- *Are my hips square, or do I usually stand more to one side, putting my weight on one foot?*
- *Are my hips, knees, and ankles aligned or do I usually turn one or both feet in or out?*

There is nothing wrong with any of these stances, after all, our bodies are extremely mobile, but there might be a problem if you are in fact standing out of alignment, but feel that you are standing straight and aligned.

Turning to the side ask the following questions:

- *If I look out of the corner of my eye without turning my head, is my head straight and balanced over the center of my body, or is tilted forward or back?*

- *Is my upper back rounded or flat?*

- *Do my arms hang forward of my body?*

- *Does my lower back curve sharply inward so that my buttocks stick out and my stomach protrudes?*

- *Can I draw a straight line through my shoulder, hip, and knee joints?*

Standing in Tadasana allows you to observe your stance and see any postural problem that you might not be aware of. Once you have realigned your body, try to identify any areas of residual tension. Pay particular attention to the shoulders and neck, your stomach muscles, and your arms, hands, and fingers; the sites of old injuries are also sometimes places where muscular tension is locked into the body. If you identify an area of tension, breathe in and contract the muscle (e.g., if your shoulders are tight, shrug them as hard as you can), then let go as you breathe out.

standing postures

The standing poses are suitable as a warm-up for the later postures. They will stretch the legs, calves, and spine, and will alleviate lower back pain. They encourage a proper alignment of the joints of the legs and hips, develop balance, and tone and strengthen the muscles of the legs.

CAUTION People with high and low blood pressure should be careful with the standing poses when starting their course of yoga study. If you feel light-headed or dizzy during a pose, discontinue the exercise and adopt one of the relaxation poses, such as the Child pose (see pages 38–9).

E

tadasana—Mountain posture

1 Stand with both feet touching from the heel to the big toe, keeping your back straight and head erect, and your arms hanging by your sides with palms facing inward.

2 To balance your weight evenly on both feet, rock gently backward and forward, finding the point of balance at the center. Your leg, buttock, and stomach muscles should be in a state of alertness—not so relaxed that you slump, but not so tensed that you cannot relax. Hold your spine in a neutral position, making sure that your lower back is not arched and that your shoulders are not rounded.

3 Tadasana is not the "standing to attention" of the soldier, which, although it may look smart and confident, is an unnatural position, because the chest is thrown out, the shoulders are too far back and out of alignment with the hips and knees, and the stomach muscles are contracted, impeding the breath.

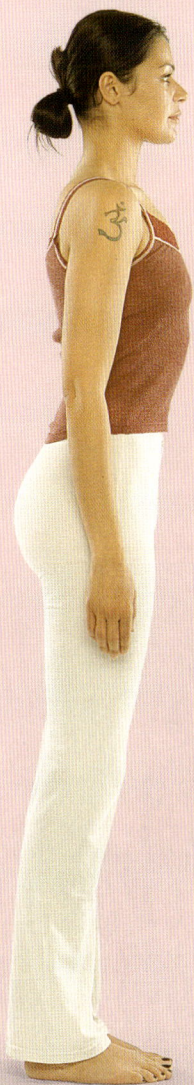

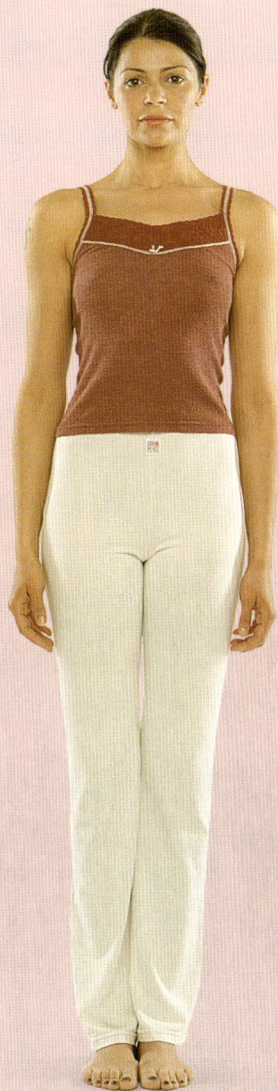

virabhadrasana I

Warrior posture

1 Stand in Tadasana. Breathe in and jump or spread your legs about four feet apart. Turn your rear foot out, making sure that your feet are on the same line.

2 Breathe out, raise your arms over your head, palms of the hands joined. Look forward or up at your hands. Hold and repeat on the other side.

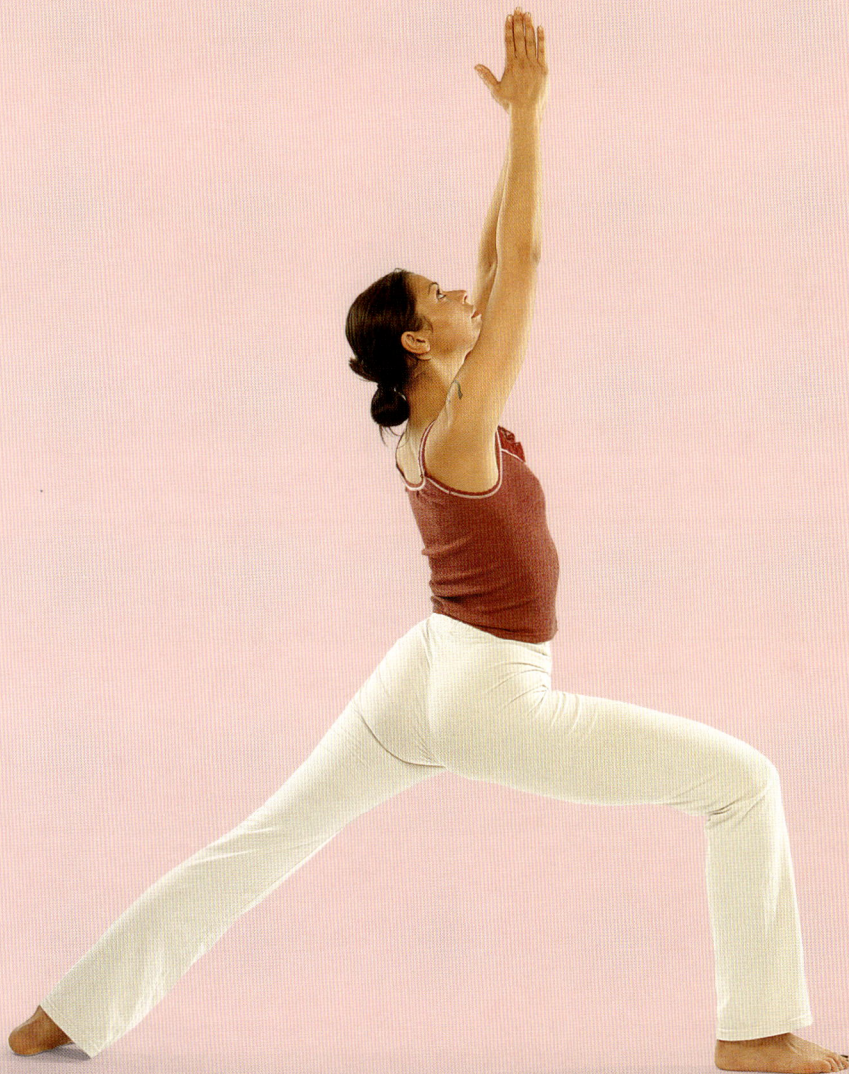

E

virabhadrasana II

Warrior II posture

1 Stand in Tadasana. Breathe in and jump or spread your legs about four feet apart. Turn your rear foot out with your feet on the same line.

2 Breathe out, raise your arms forming a straight line from the shoulders, and look at the fingers of the leading hand. Hold and repeat on the other side.

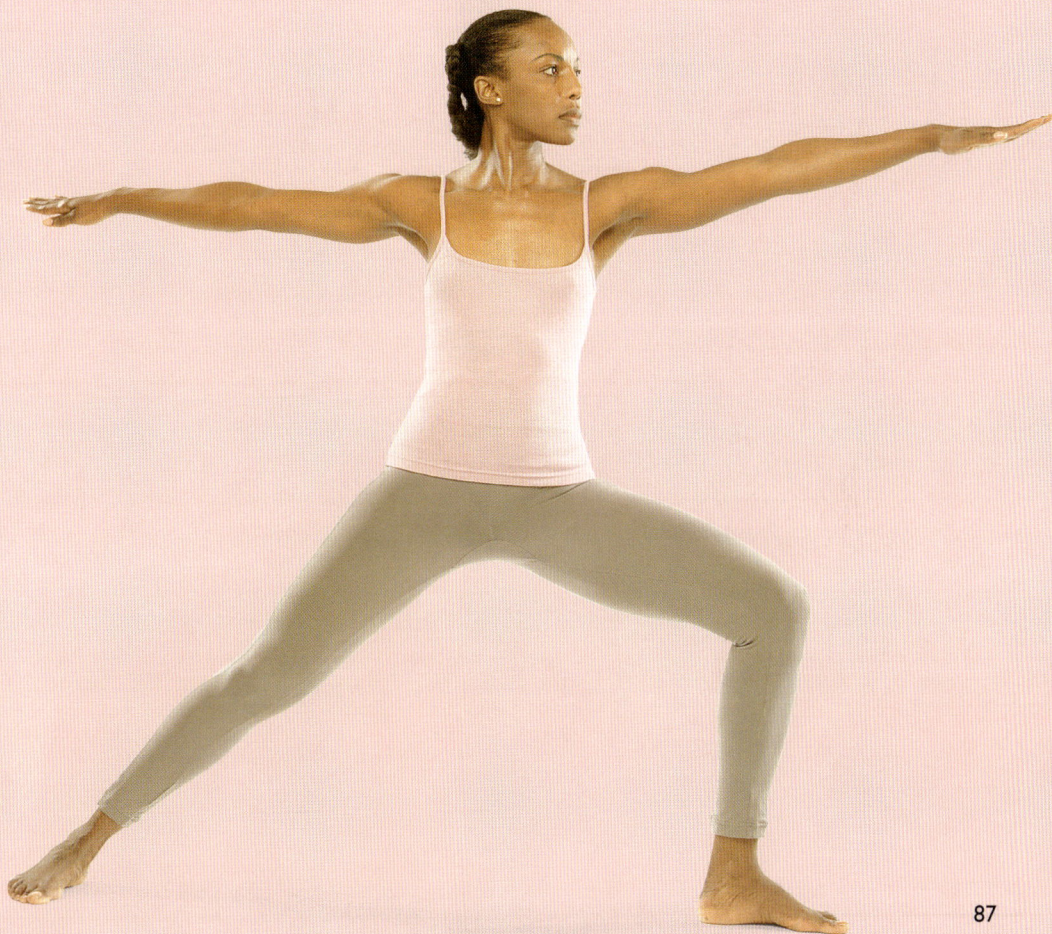

M

MEDIUM POSTURE

utthita parsvakonasana

Extended angle posture

1 Stand in Tadasana. Breathe in and jump or spread your legs about four feet apart. Extend your arms straight out from the shoulders, parallel to the floor, with the palms of your hands facing down.

2 Breathe out and turn your right foot out. Bend your left knee so that it makes a right angle.

3 Place the palm of your left hand flat on the floor next to the outside of your right foot. Your right elbow touches the outside of your right knee.

4 Stretch your right arm over your head, parallel with the floor, with the inside of the elbow over your ear. Hold, breathe in, return to a standing position, and repeat on the other side.

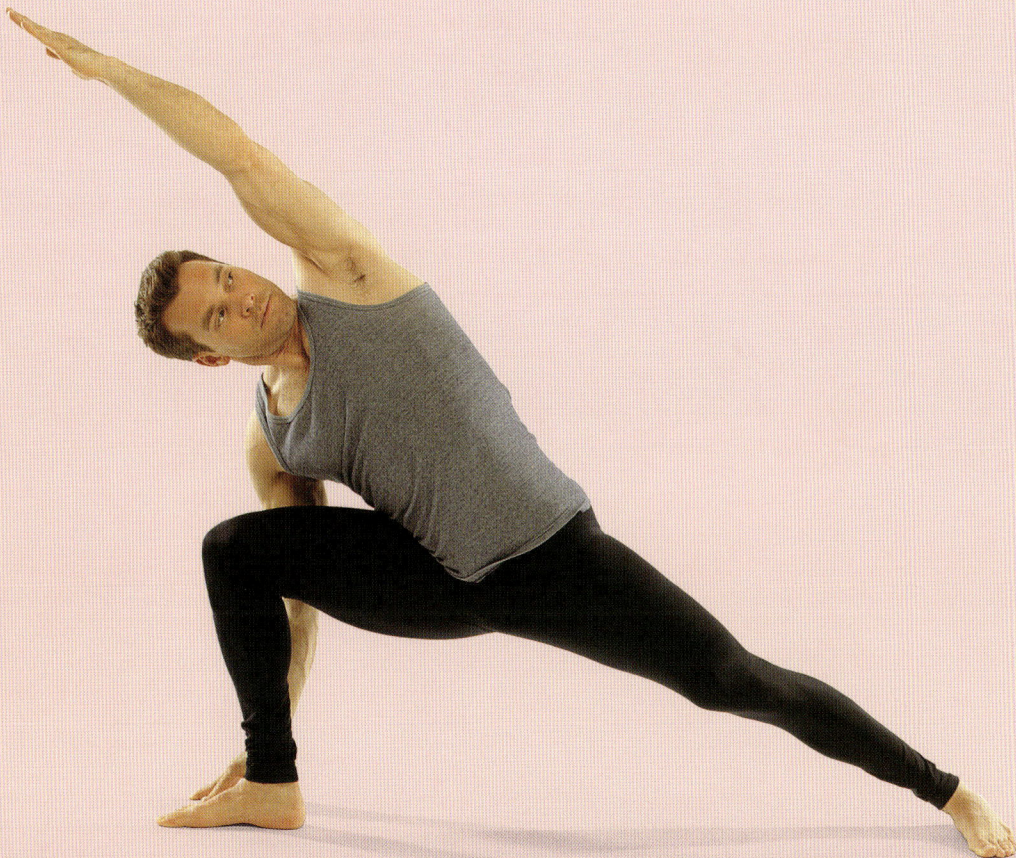

M

trikonasana—Triangle pose

1 Stand in Tadasana. Jump or step about three feet apart. Breathe in and extend both arms to the side, keeping them parallel to the floor, palms facing down. Turn your left foot out.

2 Breathe out and turn your torso to the left. Keeping your knees straight, bend at the waist and bring your left hand, palm down, next to your left ankle (or on your foot or calf if you cannot reach the floor).

3 Extend your right arm directly upward and turn your head to look at it. Hold, breathe in, return to the center and repeat on the right side.

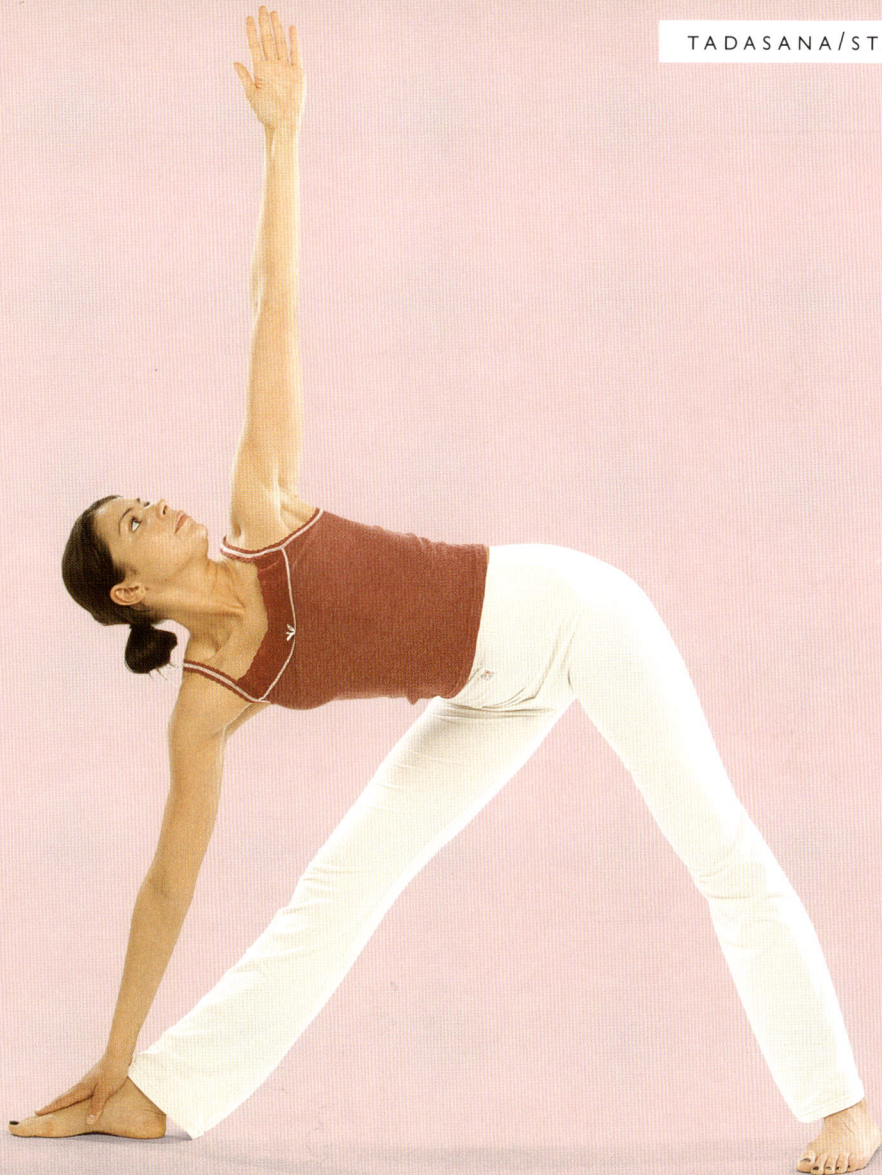

M

parsvottanasana

Forward stretch posture

1 Stand in Tadasana. Clasp your elbows behind you, or if you have good arm flexibility, in the reverse prayer position (as shown here). Breathe in and jump or walk your feet three feet apart.

2 Breathe out, and on your next in-breath turn your body to the face the right, turning your lead foot to point directly forward, and your rear foot out.

3 Breathe in, stretch up, and bend forward from the hips (and not the waist), aiming to touch your knees with your chin. Try to keep the back flat as you descend, even if means that you cannot go down as far. Hold and repeat on the other side.

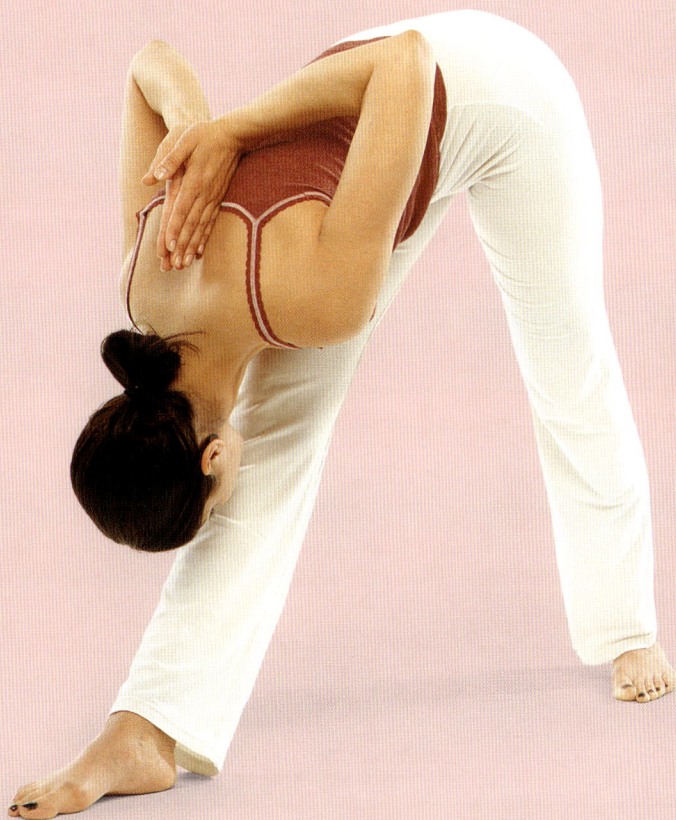

History of Yoga in the West

The first recorded contact between Westerners and yoga dates back to the fourth century BCE, when the Macedonian army of Alexander the Great (356-323 BCE) reached northern India. His troops reported seeing groups of "gymnastic holy men," but being soldiers rather than philosophers, they left no record of the yoga beliefs and practices of the time.

For a brief time during the reigns of Alexander and his immediate successors, there existed a unified empire stretching from Greece to India, permitting the untrammelled exchange of artistic, scientific, and philosophical ideas. Alexander's empire, however, quickly collapsed into warring factions after his death, and non-Hellenistic peoples overran its eastern provinces. After the rise of Islam in the seventh century, direct contact with the East was only restored in the Age of Navigation in the sixteenth century.

The arrival of Westerners in India—starting with the Portuguese, who were quickly followed by the Dutch, French, and British—did not herald any interest in Hindu religion and philosophy. Neither the rigidly Catholic French and Portuguese nor the Protestant British and Dutch, had the tolerance or breadth of vision to admit that any other religion but their own might be a valid path to salvation. Even when India was ruled by the British, interest in yoga was long limited to descriptions of "fakeers" and "heathen native practices."

The Upanishads, which have been described as the Hindu equivalent of the New Testament (see page 242), were translated into French at the beginning of the nineteenth century, attracting immediate attention from Western intellectuals. However, the history of yoga in the West really begins at the end of the century, when the first yogis travelled to Britain and the United States, first to demonstrate yoga techniques, and later to teach them.

The end of the nineteenth and the beginning of the twentieth centuries were a period of great intellectual opening in the West. In every field—art, religion, and science—new ideas swept away the fossilized edifice of Victorian certainties. At the Parliament of Religions held in Chicago in 1893, Swami Vivekananda became the first Indian yogi to make a lasting impression on the American public. Several teachers followed him, including the author of *The Autobiography of a Yogi*, Paramahansa Yogananda, who arrived in Boston in 1920. Five years later, he established the Self-Realization Fellowship in Los Angeles. Interest continued to grow, and a small number of Western students traveling to study in Indian Ashrams. Teachers continued to arrive, including the enigmatic Krishnamurti, who was groomed by the Theosophical Society as the new Messiah, but renounced this role, and whose circle included the writers George Bernard Shaw, Aldous Huxley, and Christopher Isherwood, and actor, Charlie Chaplin.

After World War Two, the head-on collision of the "counter-culture" generation with Eastern philosophies, including yoga, gave birth to the Flower Power movement and the hippies, who turned to the East in search of spiritual truths. What had been an trickle became a flood, as thousands went to India.

The ashrams and gurus, aware of the enormous potential in the spiritually starved West, began to organize themselves on corporate lines. Among the most famous gurus of the sixties were the Maharishi Mahesh Yogi and Shrila Prabhupada. The Maharishi, who won fame from his association with The Beatles, went on to create a meditative technique that he called Transcendental Meditation (TM). Prabhupada, an exponent of Bhakti yoga (yoga of devotion), founded the International Society for Krishna Consciousness (ISKCON), now a worldwide organization whose devotees can be seen chanting in the streets of major Western cities. Bhagavan Rajneesh was a more controversial, but for a time, very popular guru in the seventies and eighties whose followers became known for their alleged sexual excesses. The greatest growth in yoga, however, was in Hatha yoga, of which several major styles are now taught in the West.

Hatha yoga taught in the West

VINIYOGA

The greatest modern exponent of Hatha yoga was Sri Krishnamacharya, whose Viniyoga emphasizes practicing a posture according to one's individual needs and capacity. The regulation of breathing is an important aspect of the style, and the breath is carefully co-ordinated with the move-ments. Sri Krishnamacharya died in 1989 and was succeeded by his son, T. K. V. Desikachar.

IYENGAR

B.K.S. Iyengar is a student of Sri Krishnamacharya, who has created one of the most widely practiced styles of Hatha yoga in the West. He is the author of the best-selling *Light on Yoga* (1966). This style is characterized by slow precision perfor-mance and the aid of various props, such as cushions, chairs, wood blocks, and straps. Iyengar has trained thousands of teachers, many of whom are in the United States. His students include the late Yehudi Menuhin.

ASHTANGA

Another student of Sri Krishnamacharya, Pattabhi Jois created a style of yoga that has been adopted by such entertainers as Madonna and Julia Roberts. A "muscular" style of yoga, it teaches its own version of the Surya Namaskar, the Sun Salutation, and set series of postures. It is not to be confused with the Ashtanga yoga described in Patanjali's Yoga Sutra (see page 48).

SHIVANANDA

The yoga style that bears the name of Swami Shivananda, a former doctor who retired to the Himalayas, was created by one of his students, Swami Vishnudevananda, who opened the Shivananda Yoga Vedanta Center in Montreal in 1959, the first of many Shivananda centers world-wide. This style includes a set series of 12 postures, the Surya Namaskar, the Sun Salutation sequence, pranayama, relaxation, and mantra chanting (see page 234).

INTEGRAL

Developed by Swami Satchidananda, another student of Swami Shivananda. Satchidananda is famous for his appearance at the Woodstock music festival in 1969. This style aims to integrate the various aspects of the body-mind through a combination of postures, pranayama techniques, deep relaxation, and meditation.

KRIPALU

Kripalu yoga, inspired by Kripalvananda and developed by his disciple Yogi Amrit Desai, is a three-stage yoga created specifically for Western students. Stage one emphasizes postural alignment and co-ordination of breath and movement, with postures held for a short duration only. Stage two includes meditation, with postures held for prolonged periods. The final stage comprises "meditation in motion."

ANANDA

This style is based in the teachings of Paramahansa Yogananda, who taught in the United States in the early part of the twentieth century. It was developed by one of his disciples, Swami Kriyananda. A gentle style designed to prepare the student for meditation, it includes techniques to consciously direct prana into different parts of the body.

BIKRAM

Bikram Choudhury, who achieved fame as the teacher of Hollywood stars, teaches at the Yoga College of India in Bombay. His system of 26 postures are performed in a standard sequence in a room heated to 100–110°F. This approach is fairly vigorous and requires a high degree of physical fitness on the part of participating students.

KUNDALINI

This style of Hatha yoga, created by the Sikh master Yogi Bhajan, aims to awaken the spiritual energy stored at the base of the spine, by means of postures, pranayama, mantra chanting, and meditation.

Timeline

Increasingly popular in the West, yoga has its roots in ancient India. The migration of yoga from East to West has taken place over 150 years. The map and time line provided here illustrate this migration, pinpointing some of the key locations where yoga was established in the US.

5,000 year old ceramics from the ancient cities of Mojendro-Daro and Harappa in Indus Valley on the Indian subcontinent depict yoga positions. The evolution from a contemporary animist religion is evident in the many yoga asanas named after animals and nature: cobra, tree, mountain, dog, camel, crocodile and peacock.

3,000 B.C.E stone seals showing figures in yogic postures excavated from the Indus valley. These yogic postures resemble Lord Shiva and Parvathi performing various Asanas and practicing meditation. According to mythical tradition, Shiva is said to be the founder of yoga, and Paravati his first disciple.

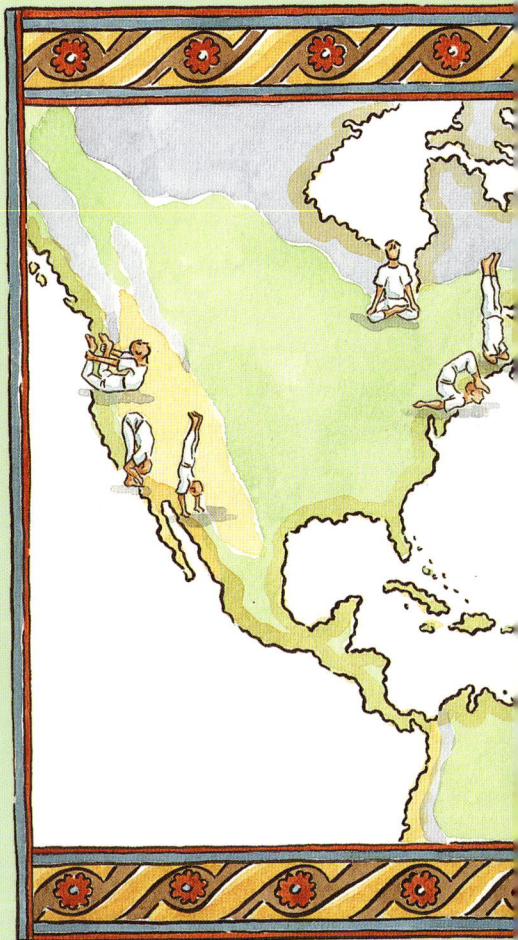

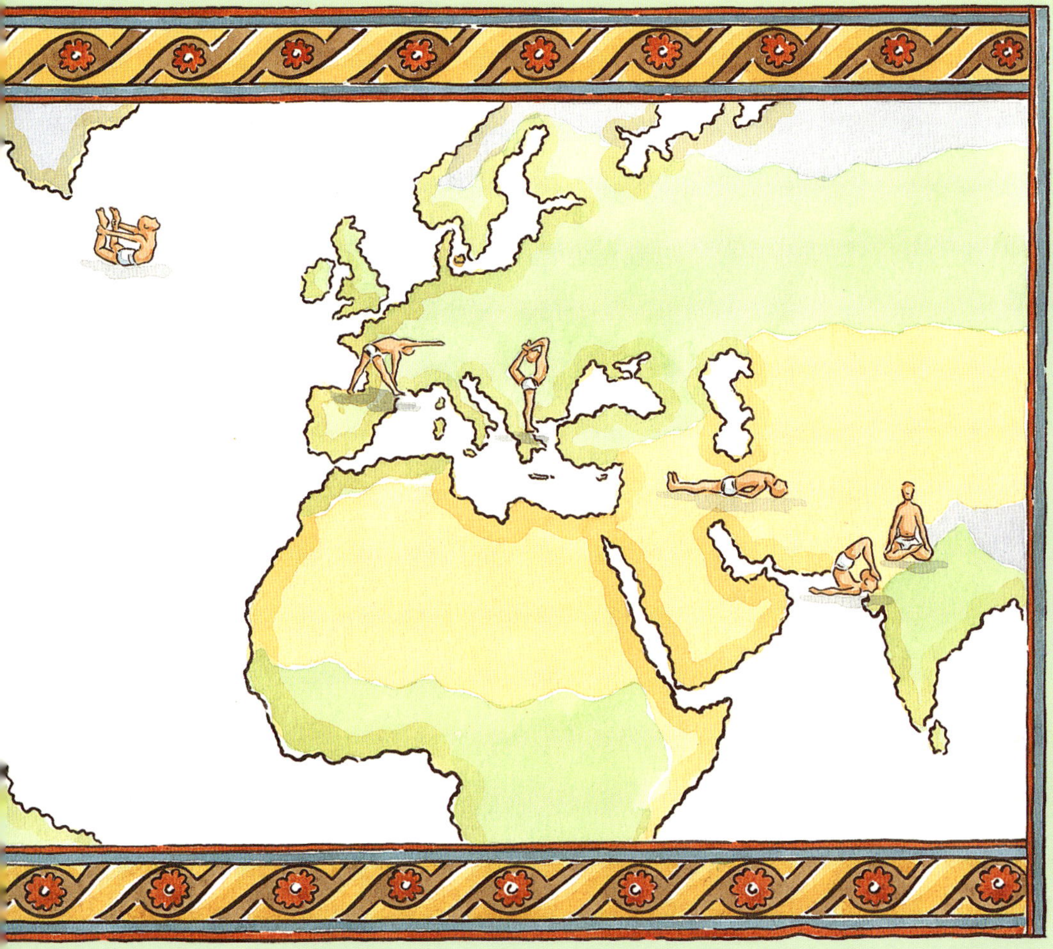

2,500 B.C.E. A vast collection of scriptures called the Vedas were recorded. Rig Veda, Sama Veda and Yajur Veda were a collection of 1008 hymns on theology, social institutions, legal systems, ethics, cosmology, philosophy and science. *The Rig Veda* is considered an authoritative sacred work by the Hindu faith.

800–600 B.C.E. Upanishads written, providing the main foundation of yoga teaching. "Upanishad" means "teachings received by a pupil sitting before a sage via a lineage of Masters" and is still a popular means for transmitting yogic knowledge. Over 200 Upanishads exist but only 10–12 are considered the most authoritative.

300 B.C.E. *The Bhagavad Gita* (the Song of the Blessed Lord), written by Sage Vyasa is a spiritual poem and a treatise on yoga, especially Bhakti, Jnana and Karma. The "Gita" is part of the great eight-chapter epic called the Mahabharata compiled by many authors over hundreds of years; the latter takes the form of a discourse delivered by Krishna (the Lord) to Arjuna (the hero) expounding on the ultimate goal of life.

500 B.C.E. and the early Christian era, Jainism and Buddhism became more popular in the East. While they contained elements of yoga in them, both rejected the Vedas. Buddhism was strong in the 3rd century BC, but Orthodox Hinduism which evolved from the Vedas, overtook its popularity. Eventually around the 7th century Buddhism left for other lands.

200–800 B.C.E. Patanjali detailed the entire sum of knowledge about yoga in 196 aphorisms (sutras), referred to also as Raja yoga. Patanjali is part of the classical yoga era, when thousands of yoga asanas were still being practiced. *The Yoga Sutras of Patanjali* is considered the authoritative text on classical yoga by all yoga schools and used by many contemporary yoga styles.

600–1200 A.D. Tantrism developed in India from the esoteric teachings of sects and brotherhoods. It is reflected in countless images of Mithuna—embracing couples—which adorn Hindu temples. The Tantras, written during the Middle Ages, were sacred poems that included instruction on ceremonies.

c. 1200–1850 The main branches of yoga were established. The sacred writings such as the *Hatha yoga Pradipika*, *Yogatattva*, *yoga Yajnavalkya*, *Puranas*, *Shrimad Bhagavatam*, *Gherunda Samhita*, and *Siva Samhita* and their interpretations detail the practices for each path. The yogic paths include: Jnana (union by knowledge), Karma (by action), Bhakti (by devotion), Raja (by mind mastery), Tantra (by sexual energy), Kundalini (by serpent power), Yantra (by symbols), Mantra (by sound) and Kriya (by several practices).

c. 1850 The more contemplative stages—Raja and Jnana yoga—initially ignited the interest of an exclusive group of Americans. Referring to themselves as transcendentalists, an elite group of intellectuals known as the Concord Circle, and including Ralph Waldo Emerson and Henry David Thoreau drew inspiration from the Bhagavad Gita. Thus were the seeds for the growth of yoga in America planted.

1875 Colonel Henry Steel Olcott, a prominent New York lawyer, and Helene Blavatsky, a Russian emigré and occultist, established the Theosophical Society in New York City. Blavatsky, as renowned for being a cigar-smoking eccentric as she was for her esoteric knowlege, went on to publish two important works, *Isis Unveiled* in 1877 and *The Secret Doctrine* in 1888. These two voluminous treatises collectively divulged many of the secret teachings of the ancient Vedic texts.

1893 Swami Vivekananda arrives to address the World Parliament of Religions in Chicago, Illinois. Vivekananda lectured on the merits of Raja yoga, a theme he would reiterate often during his two-year stay in the United States.

1899 Vivekananda returned again to America where he founded the New York Vedanta Society, a thriving community that focuses on four of the six branches of yoga: raja, karma, bhakti, and jnana.

1919 Yogendra Mastamani landed in Long Island. He began to demonstrate the power of Hatha yoga to Northeastern America. Before Mastamani left the United States in 1922, he founded the first American branch of Kaivalyadhama, establishing yoga as a viable healing therapy. His connection with Benedict Lust, the founder of naturopathy, began a relationship between yoga and alternative medicine and healing practices that continues today.

1920–1925 Paramahansa Yogananda arrives in Boston to address the International Congress of Religious Liberals. After a three-year tenure in Boston, Yogananda toured the United States and wound up in Los Angeles where he founded the Self Realization Fellowship (SRF). SRF has attracted hundreds of thousands of followers throughout the years and remains a strong force within the yoga community. Yogananda's *Autobiography of a Yogi* (1946) turned an entire generation of seekers on to yoga and Eastern spirituality.

1947 Latvian-born Indra Devi, known as the "First Lady of Yoga" in America, set down roots in Hollywood, California, and opened her first U.S. yoga studio. Hollywood luminaries quickly embraced her teachings and she is credited with almost single-handedly establishing a niche for American Hatha yoga.

1961 Richard Hittleman's TV show sets Americans about practicing yoga in front of their TV sets in droves. The medium of television provided a venue through which millions more could learn this ancient discipline. Hittleman wrote among his many other books, *The Twenty-Eight-Day Yoga Plan*, which sold millions of copies.

1968 Ananda Village, a 750-acre spread in Nevada City, California, was founded by Swami Kriyananda, an American disciple of Paramahansa Yogananda. In response to the growing need for spiritual awakening, gurus—both foreign and domestic—sprung up all over America, and whole communities were established along with them.

1960s and 1970s The social and political climate created a free-spirited individualism that encouraged people of all ages to question and explore their values. This exploration led to an intense interest in Asian cultures and exotic philosophies. Fueled by The Beatles' much publicized visit to India, and their initiation into Maharishi Mahesh Yogi's Transcendental Meditation—along with the publication of Ram Dass's *Be Here Now*—meditation became *de rigeur*.

Late 1970s Baba Hari Dass founded Mt. Madonna near Santa Cruz, California, and Swami Satchidananda's Yogaville established roots in Buckingham, Virginia. A distinctly American brand of Hatha yoga also began to evolve during this time, with the arrival of several visiting yoga teachers from India. Yogi Bhajan, B.K.S. Iyengar, and Swami Vishnu-devananda all made an indelible mark on the landscape of American yoga, each bringing a distinct style of Hatha yoga to the attention of eager students.

"If a wise man holds his chest, neck, and head even, and turns his senses inward toward his heart, he will be able to cross the torrents of fear in the boat of Brahman."

Svetasvatara Upanishad

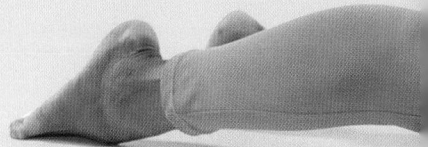

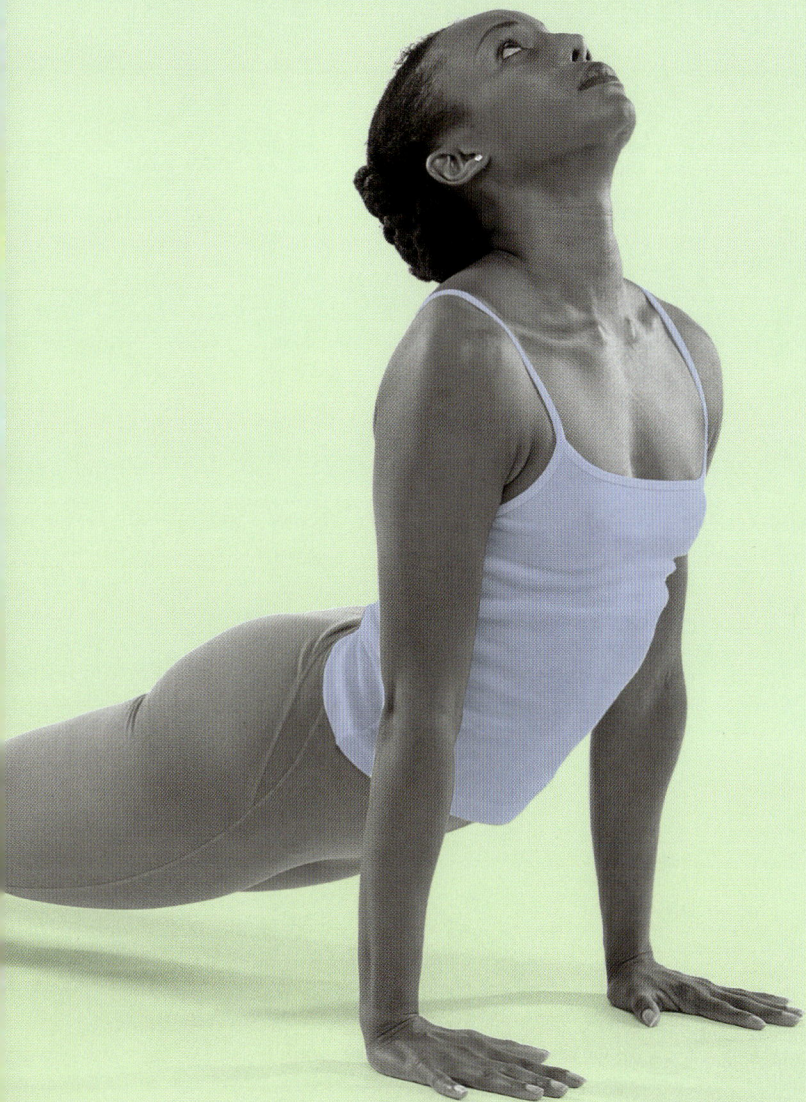

vrakasana

balance

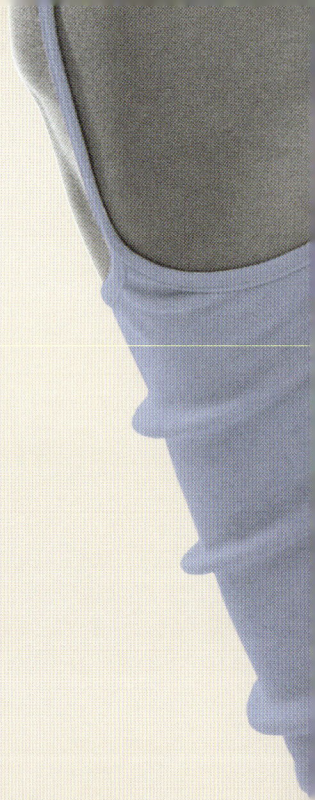

Vrksa means tree. A tree is firmly rooted in the earth, but it is also flexible and can bend in the wind.

chapter 4

benefits

Balance is not a skill that many of us will train once we are past childhood. Like all other physical skills, balance is subject to the "use it or lose it" principle. The primary physical benefit of Vrksasana is that it allows you to practice your balancing skills. It also strengthens and tones the legs, as the entire weight of the body rests on one leg at a time.

The benefits of Vrksasana, however, are not limited to the purely physical. A yoga teacher I know once told me that she practices Vrksasana when she needs to focus all her attention on a difficult mental task, such as doing her accounts. Unless you have an impairment of the organs of balance located in your ears, poor balance is not a physical problem but one of distracted attention. The regular practice of Vrksasana will help improve your powers of concentration. In my personal practice, I find that when I can effortlessly hold Vrksasana, it gives me a sense of self-confidence and achievement.

balancing postures

Balance is not a skill that is developed only in the legs. As we see in the following asanas, this includes postures balancing on your hands and in a seated position. These will develop strength and tone in the arm and abdominal muscles. As a beginner you may find several of the asanas quite strenuous. As in the inverted postures, make sure that the area around you is clear of obstacles and breakable objects you might fall on. A yoga teacher once admitted to me that she had destroyed her television set when she fell on it while attempting a balance pose as a beginner. Like Vrksasana, all the balancing asanas will help you develop your powers of concentration.

E

vrksasana—Tree posture

1 Stand in Tadasana. To aid your concentration before starting the exercise, take several deep breaths and fix your gaze on a point directly in front of you.

2 Breathe in and bend your right leg at the knee, then raise your right foot as high up the inside of your left thigh as possible. If you have good ankle flexibility, place the upper part of your right foot on top of your thigh, sole facing outward.

3 You may be unsteady at the beginning. Breathe deeply and sink into your supporting leg. When you are ready, breathe in and raise both arms above the head, palms together.

4 Breathe out, lower your arms and right leg and return to Tadasana. Repeat on the other side.

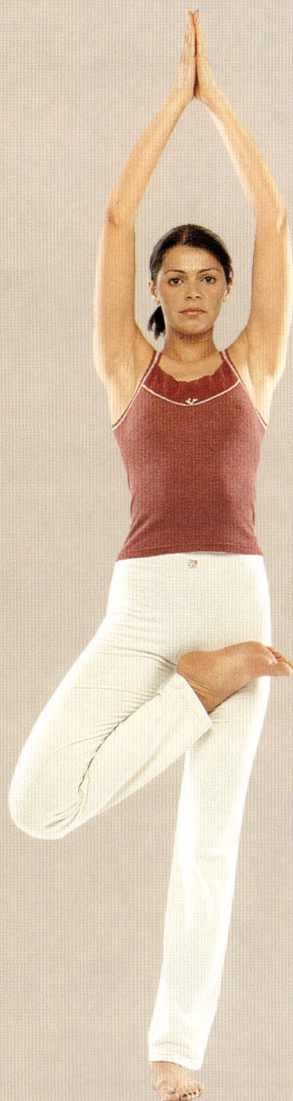

III

kakasana—Crow posture

1 Squat on your toes with your knees apart. Breathe out and place your palms between your knees on the floor, shoulder-width apart, fingers spread (figure 1).

2 Breathe in and place the inner edge of your knees on the backs of your upper arms (figure 2).

3 Lift your legs off the floor (together or singly) until you are balanced on your hands. Look forward while keeping your elbows slightly bent (figure 3).

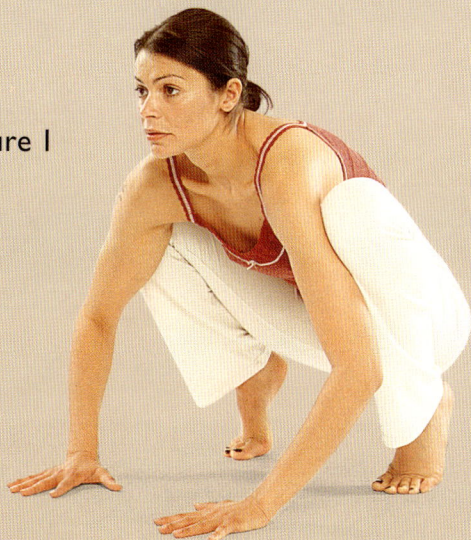

figure 1

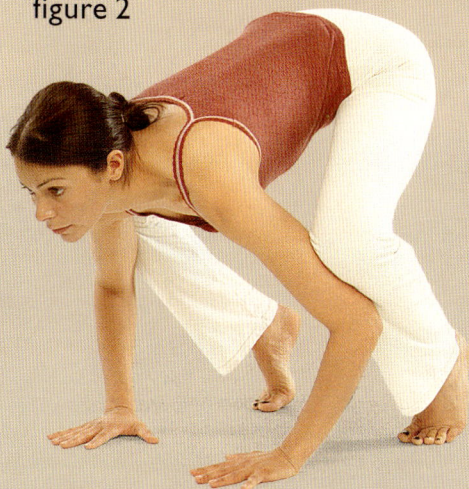

figure 2

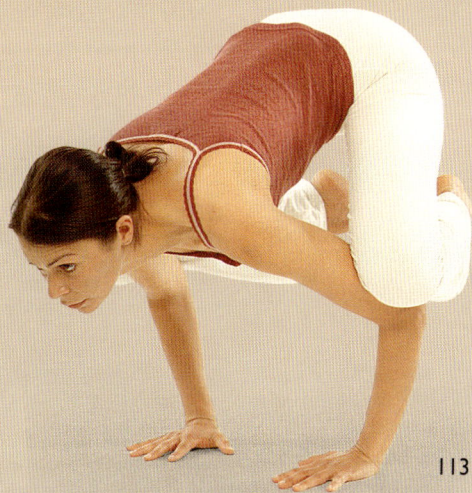

figure 3

113

M

utthita padangusthasana

One leg balance posture

1 Stand in Tadasana. As in the tree posture, fix a spot in front of you with your gaze to aid concentration, and take several deep breaths to settle yourself.

2 Breathe out as you bend your right leg and catch hold of your big toe with the thumb and first two fingers of your right hand. Breathe in and place your left hand on your left hip.

3 When you are ready, breathe out and stretch your leg. Try to keep your supporting leg and back straight, and raise your right leg as high as possible. Hold and repeat with the left leg.

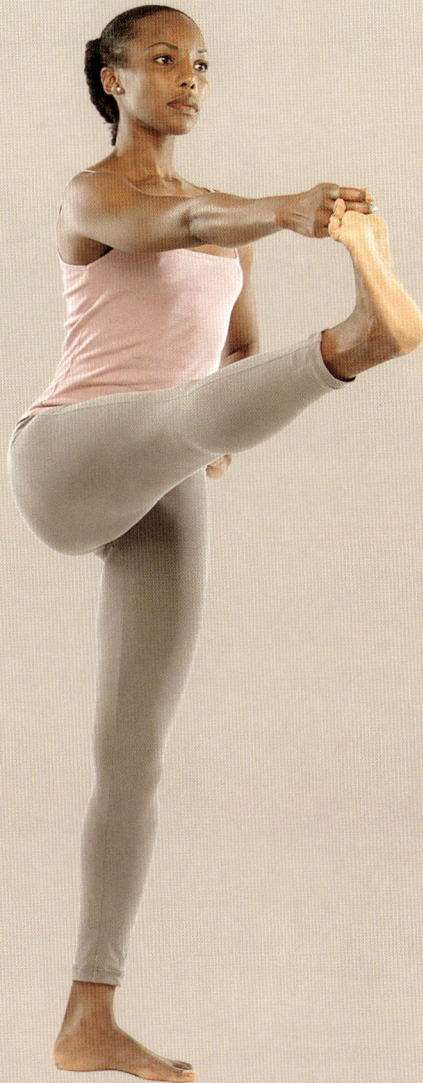

ubhaya padangusthasana

Sitting balance posture

1 Sit on the floor with your legs outstretched, feet together. Breathe out, bend your knees and hold your big toes with your thumb and first two fingers. Hold this position until you are balanced.

2 Breathe in, stretch your legs and arms, and balance on your buttocks so that your body makes the shape of the letter V.

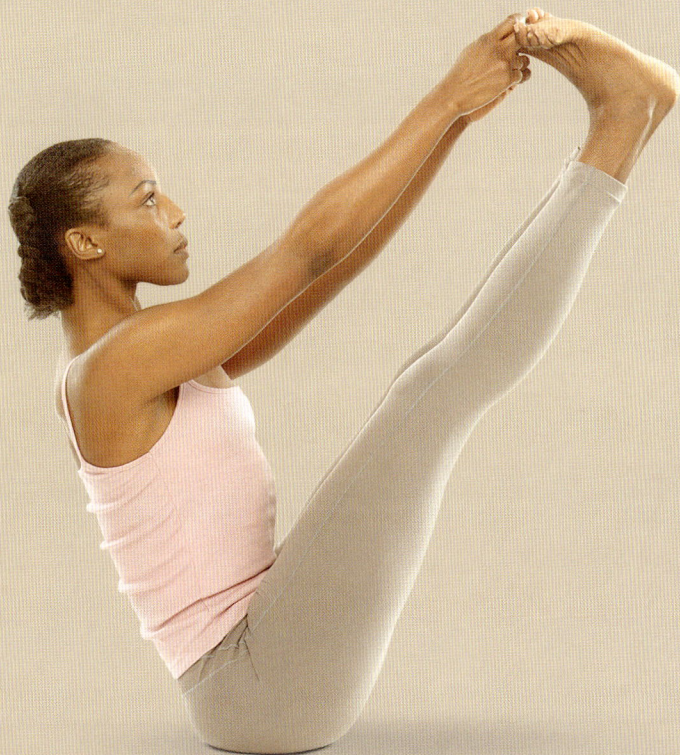

Yogic lifestyle

In traditional Hindu culture, there are four stages in the life of a male member of the Brahmin caste. As a youth he is expected to study the scriptures; as an adult to perform his priestly duties, marry, and father a family; in his maturity, to seek a spiritual path to liberation; and in his old age, to renounce the world and prepare himself for his next life. Although this pattern holds true for many yogis in India, there are also those who have renounced their caste affiliation and rejected the life and duties of an adult. Some choose to live as sadhus, or ascetics, in the forest where they practice austerities, while others live in ashrams (communities) as celibate followers of a particular guru, or teacher.

The lifestyle of the yogi, whether he lives alone or in a community is governed by a set of strict moral commandments.

These are explained in the Hatha Yoga Pradipika in the following verse:

"Not to cause suffering to any living creature; to speak the truth; not to steal or covet the things of others; to practice continence; to develop compassion and fortitude; to be merciful to all; to be moderate in eating. These are the first prerequisites to yoga.

Self discipline, cheerfulness, faith, charity, contemplation, listening to sacred scriptures, a clean mind, recitation of mantras, and observance of rules, these are the second requirements of yoga."

A slightly more relaxed set of rules applies to students of yoga who are married or partnered. In this case, there is no prohibition against sexual relations or living in your own home and raising your family.

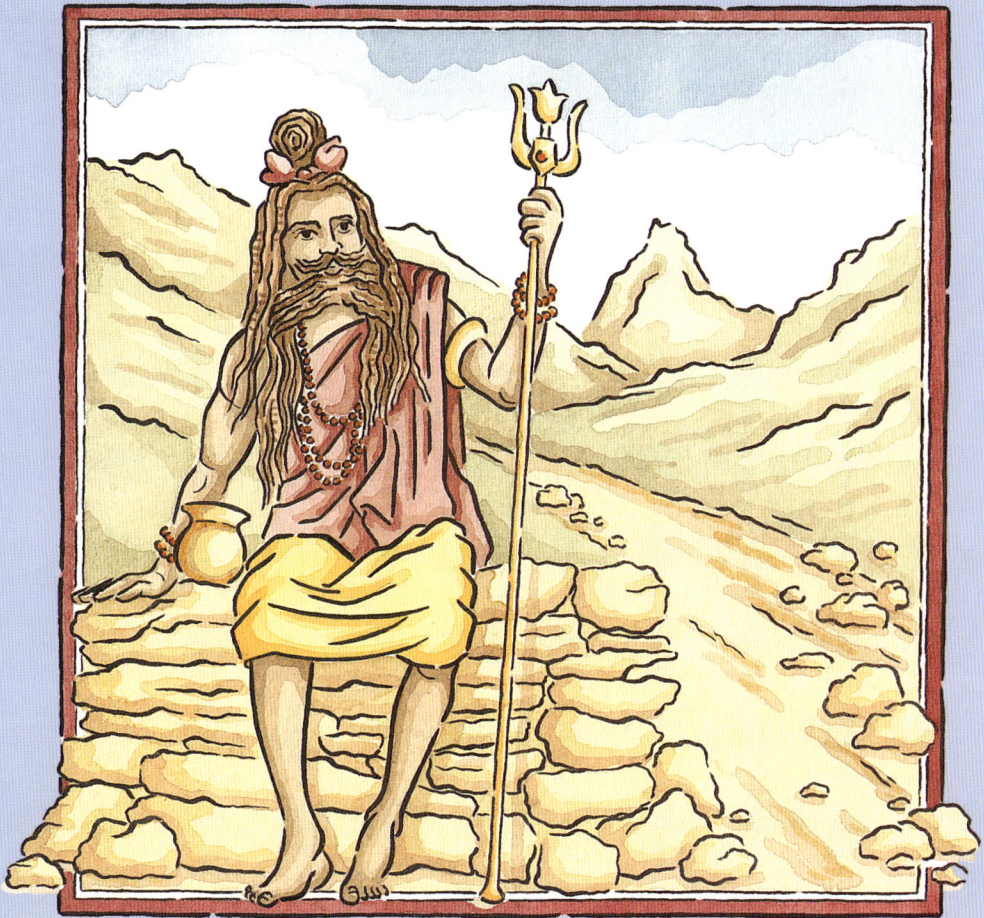

Yogic hygiene

Purity of the body is no less important than purity of the mind, and the yogic lifestyle enjoins cleansing practices that go far beyond brushing one's teeth and cleaning one's skin and hair by showering or bathing. In Dhauti, cleansing takes on a much broader meaning: in addition to the physical removal of external dirt or impurities, there are practices that are designed to cleanse the body internally, as well as cleansing the breath, and the pranic or astral body (see page 71).

The breath is cleansed with pranayama techniques such as Kapalabhati (see page 66) or the bellows breath, Bhastrika, in which air is pumped vigorously into and out of the lungs. These techniques are also said to generate prana (see pages 56–7).

One of the principle techniques of Dhauti is the cleansing of the stomach and the walls of the oesophagus by swallowing a long strip of cloth (nowadays, surgical gauze) soaked in salted water or milk, which is left in the stomach and then pulled out. This and other internal techniques described below should only be attempted under the supervision of a qualified teacher. In addition to stomach cleansing, Yogis practice both colonic (Vasti) and bladder irrigation (Vajroli mudra). In Vasti water is drawn into the body by muscle contraction alone, using Uddiyana bandha (see pages 74–5) and moved around with Nauli, churning the stomach muscles.

The nose and sinuses are cleaned using either a catheter or soft rope passed through the nostrils and out of the mouth, or by pouring salted water into one nostril and out of the other. In addition to the cleaning techniques for ears, throat, teeth, and tongue, yogis perform Trataka to "cleanse" the eyes. In this technique you stare at a candle flame until your eyes water, and then, closing your eyes, you picture the flame in your mind's eye.

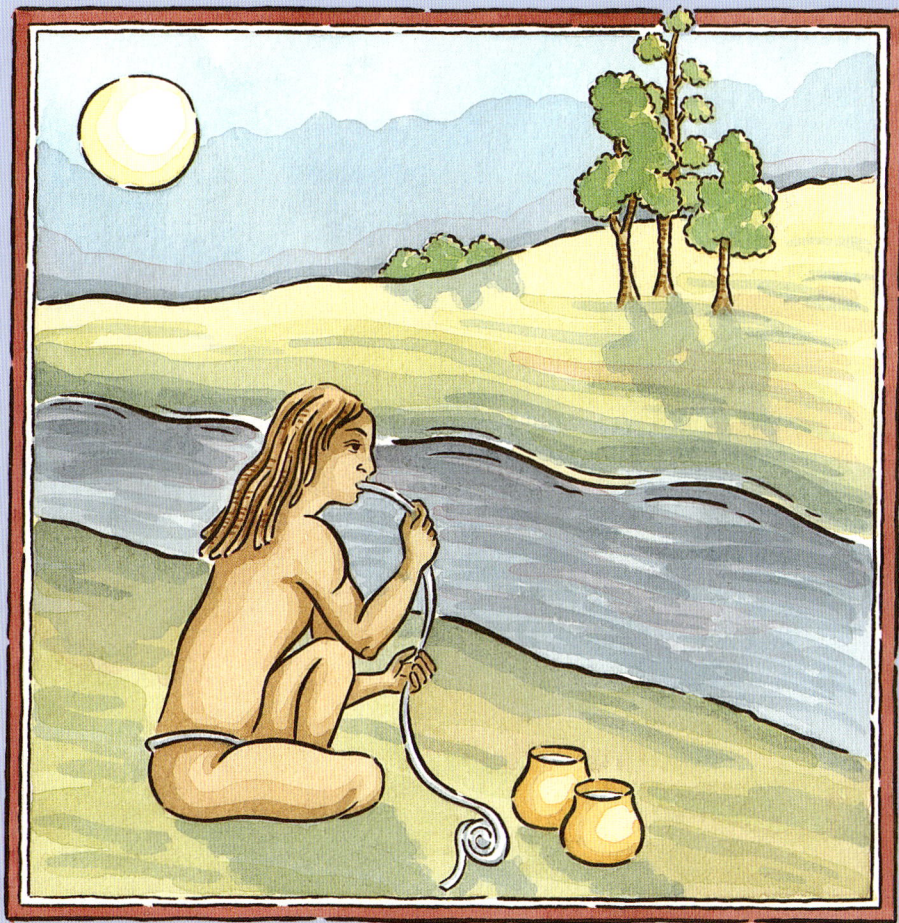

Yogic diet

Physical and mental purity is also maintained by strict attention to diet. Traditionally yogis are lacto-vegetarian; they abstain from meat and fish but include milk and certain other animal products in their diets. Yogis do not eat animal flesh for both health-related and ethical reasons. Although in the West reincarnation is often given as the reason for vegetarianism, in the East, this is an over-simplification. The main ethical reason is in the principle of Ahimsa, non-violence and non-injury to any living creature, which is one of the moral injunctions the yogi is charged to follow.

The Hatha Yoga Pradipika gives the following dietary guidelines:

"Avoid sour, pungent, and hot food, mustard, alcohol, fish, meat, curds, buttermilk, chick peas, linseed cakes, asafoetida, and garlic. It is also advisable to avoid reheated food, an excess of salt or acid, foods that are hard to digest or are woody."

And further advises, "The following foods can be eaten without hesitation: wheat products, rice, milk, fats, rock candy, honey, dried ginger, cucumbers, vegetables, and fresh water... The yogi should eat nourishing, sweet foods mixed with milk. He should benefit the senses and stimulate the bodily functions."

The categories described include three types of food: foods that are over-stimulating, such as spicy foods or coffee; foods that are believed to create inertia, such as mushrooms; reheated foods, and alcohol. The foods that are recommended in the text are said to be pure and to calm and sharpen the mind.

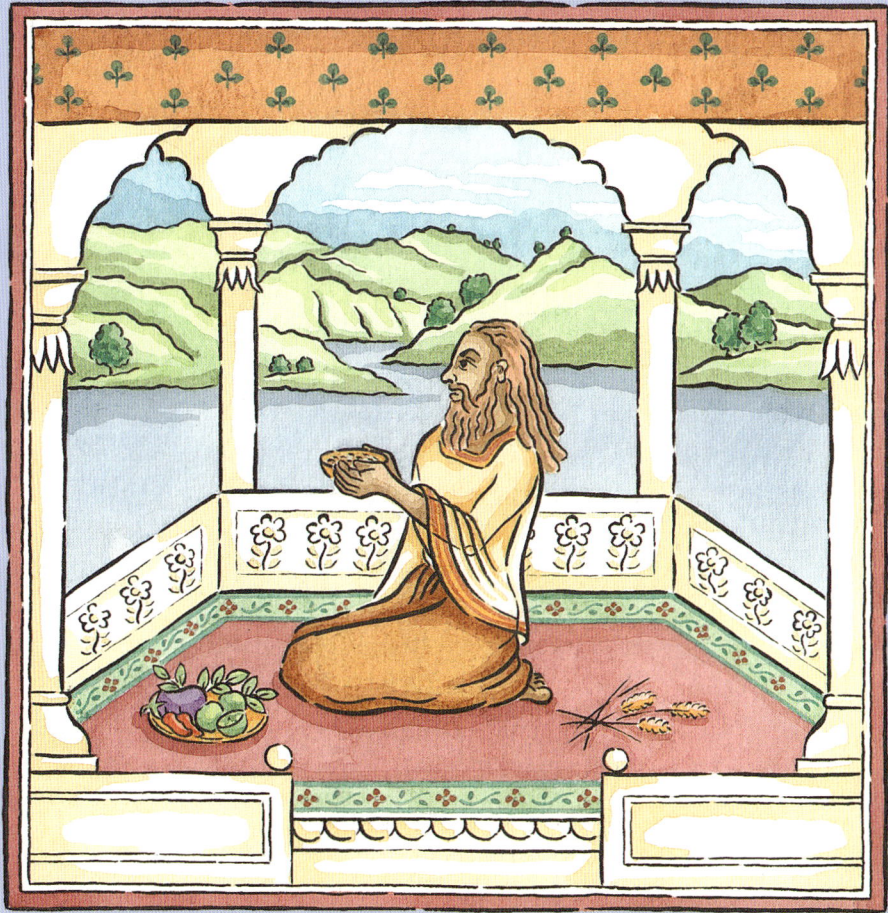

Yoga and weight-control

Many Westerners take up exercise with a view to losing weight, and yoga is no exception. My mother was one of the many middle-aged women who started yoga for this reason, and while she undoubtedly benefited from the practice of yoga in many different ways—improving her flexibility, concentration, and reducing her level of stress—she did not lose weight.

The yogi follows a strict path of self-discipline and exercise combined with the lacto-vegetarian diet and abstinence from alcohol. Devotees of this path will completely transform their physical appearance, but only because they are changing their entire lifestyles. If your main goal is weight-loss, then this may seem a rather excessive sacrifice to make. When choosing an exercise system, you have to be very certain of what you want it to do for you.

On a physical level, although yoga does develop muscular tone and endurance, especially the more "athletic" schools, such as Ashtanga and Power yoga, it will not encourage fat burning in the same way that jogging or aerobic classes do.

Yoga and longevity

Although I can only rely on personal experience rather than scientific evidence, after working for more than two decades in the health and fitness industry, I am convinced that yoga can slow the aging process.

When people begin to exercise, they suddenly seem to rejuvenate. A healthy glow to the skin from improved circulation, and greater energy levels are just two of the benefits we obtain from exercise. Yoga, however, is unique since, in addition to this, it also promotes a high degree of flexibility, and relaxation. Combined, these are the key to maintaining a body that is not simply young-looking on the outside but equally more healthy on the inside. The flexibility you develop from the practice of the asanas combats the loss of elasticity of our bodies that is a natural part of the aging process, and meditation and pranayama deal with any form of stress-related muscular tension (see page 146).

bhujangasana
bend

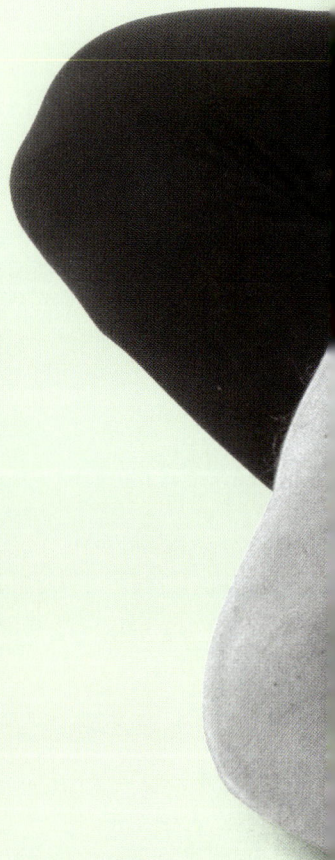

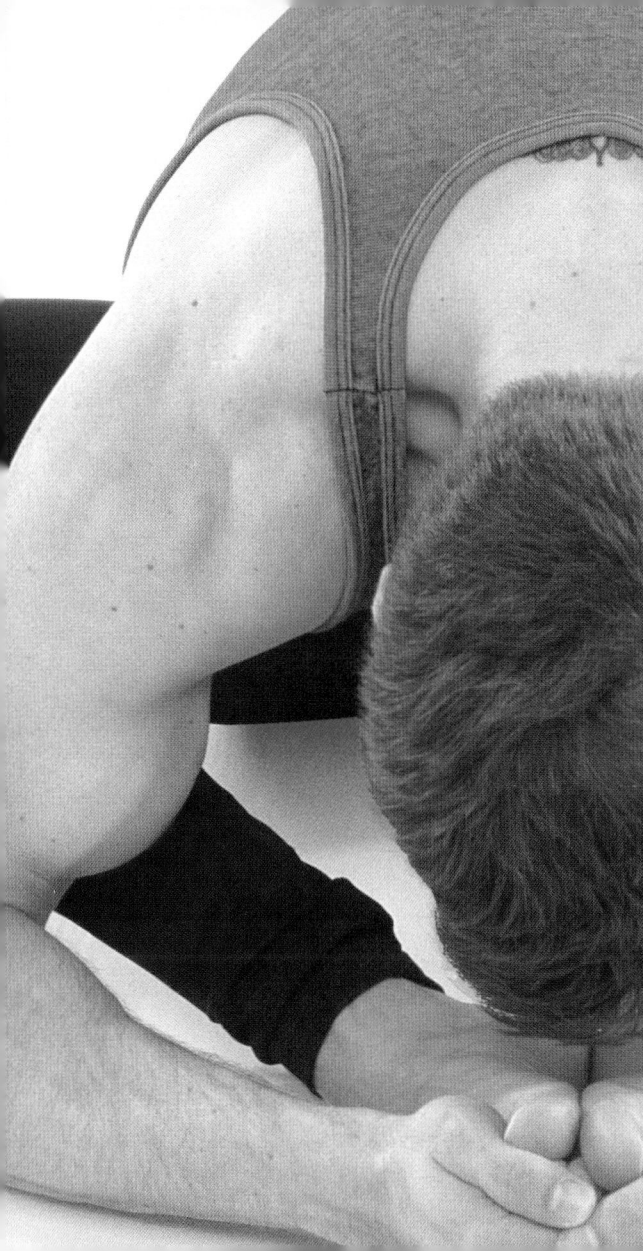

The word bhujanga means snake; it is derived from the verb root bhuj meaning to bend or curve.

chapter 5

benefits

The spine is the body's "information superhighway," carrying data from the senses to the brain, and relaying instructions from the brain to the muscles and joints. In addition to this vital role, we also often forget that the spine is the body's largest and most important joint, providing us with excellent mobility by allowing us to bend forward and backward, from side to side, and to twist around.

Western strength-training techniques immobilize the spine by encasing it in shortened, inflexible muscles that are prone to injury, a failing that I discovered to my own cost, when in my twenties, I strained my lower back during a set of heavy squats. I was laid up for a week and had to walk with crutches for several more. After regular stretching of the spine with the bending asanas, the injury has not recurred in two decades of intense physical training.

Traumatic spinal injuries that temporarily or permanently disable are extremely rare when compared to the daily plight of the millions who suffer from lower-back and neck problems, which are caused primarily by sedentary lifestyles. The first of many benefits of the bending asanas is that by stretching and strengthening the muscles of the back, they restore the flexibility of the spine and alleviate or cure many spinal problems. The stretch of the thighs in two of the postures (see the Pascimottonasana —Forward bend, pages 138–9 and Dhanurasana asanas—Bow, pages 142–3) also tackles another major cause of back pain: tight hamstrings.

In advanced practice, Bhujangasana is one of the postures used to arouse Kundalini, the spiritual energy that lies dormant at the base of the spine.

bending postures

These asanas are vital in maintaining a healthy, flexible spine, and should be practiced, if possible, on a daily basis. If you suffer from recurring lower-back pain, start with the easy (E) and medium (M) postures, and gradually build up your confidence and flexibility until you are ready for the difficult (D) postures. Stop immediately if you feel any undue back pain. If there is a structural problem in your spine, such as damage to the intervertebral disks, the postures may be dangerous, and you should consult your doctor before attempting them. Remember that when you bend your spine in one direction, you should bend it in the opposite direction to maintain a balanced stretch.

After a day working at the computer, I find that a round of bending asanas is the best medicine against any stiffness or aches and pains. I have also found that the massage of the internal organs and increased blood-flow to the body cavity improve a range of digestive problems.

"A yogi who wishes to develop siddhis should keep Hatha Yoga strictly secret, for only then will he succeed. All his efforts will be in vain if he reveals all without discrimination."

Hatha Yoga Pradipika

M

bhujangasana—Serpent posture

1 Lie on your stomach, legs extended behind you, feet together, toes pointed, with your head to one side resting on your hands, palms flat on the floor.

2 Take a long slow breath to center yourself. Lift your head, and place your hands just below your shoulders with the fingertips in line with the top of your shoulders. Place your forehead on the floor between your hands.

3 Breathe in, press down on your hands, and lift your head and upper body, pushing your hips into the floor and arching your shoulders backward. Do not allow your elbows to splay out, but keep them tight into your body.

4 Raise your head and upper body as high as is comfortable. Avoid putting pressure on your hands, and keep your elbows slightly bent so as not to hunch your shoulders. Look directly forward, or if comfortable, tilt your head back.

5 Breathe out, and return to the start position, slowly unrolling the spine.

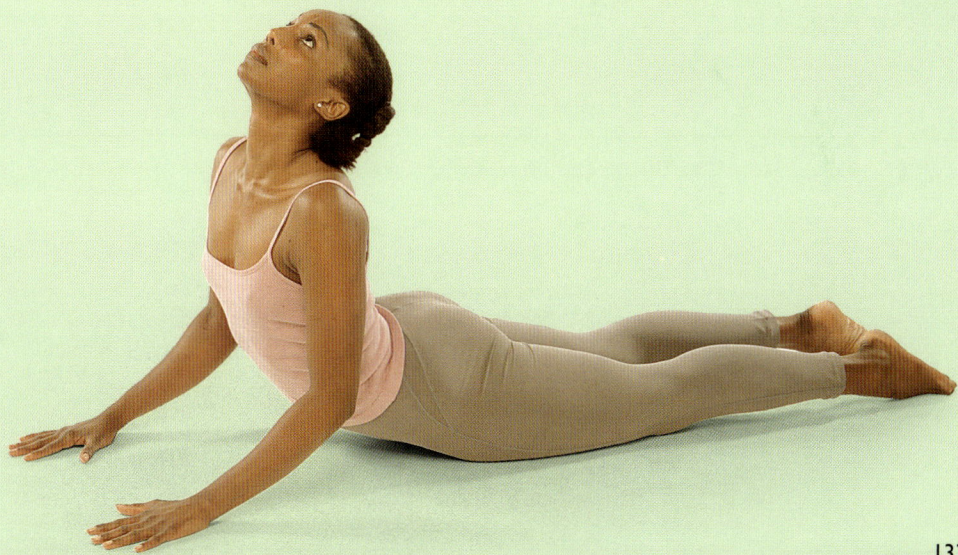

E

Cat posture

1 Kneel on all fours with your hands directly under your shoulders and your legs forming right angles with your torso. Your back is flat and holds no tension.

2 Breathe in. Push down in your lower back, and tilt your head upward, in the manner of a cat arching its back (figure 1).

3 Breathe out. Drop your head and round your back as much as possible (figure 2).

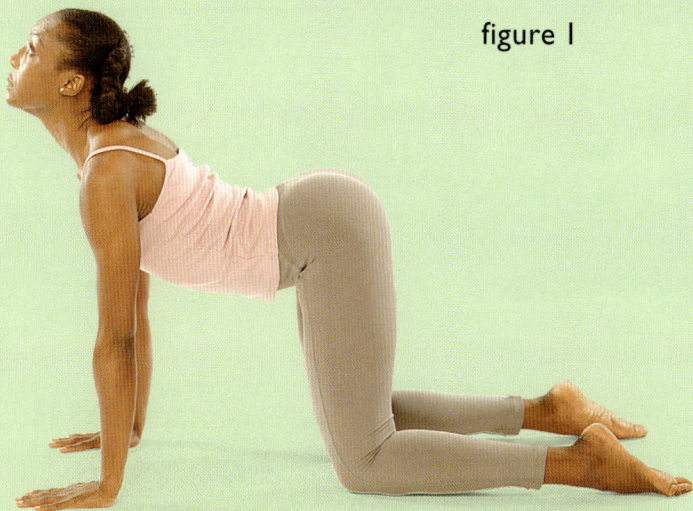

figure 1

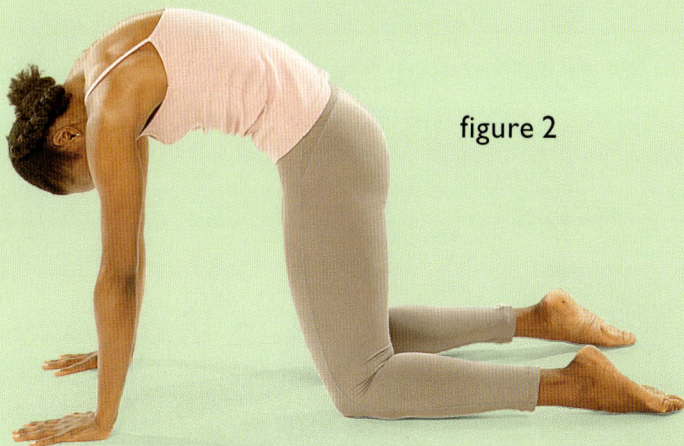

figure 2

E

EASY POSTURE

matsyasana—Fish posture

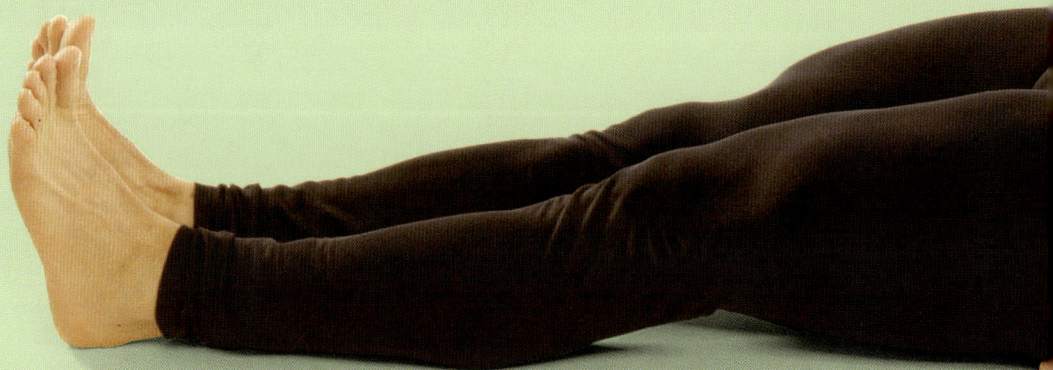

1 Lie on your back with your legs and feet together, toes pointed, and your forearms and hands by your side, with palms down under your thighs.

2 Breathe in, bend your elbows, pushing your forearms into the floor, and raise your upper body and head.

3 Breathe out, drop your head back so that it is touching the floor, but do not rest your weight on it. Make sure your knees and buttocks stay on the floor.

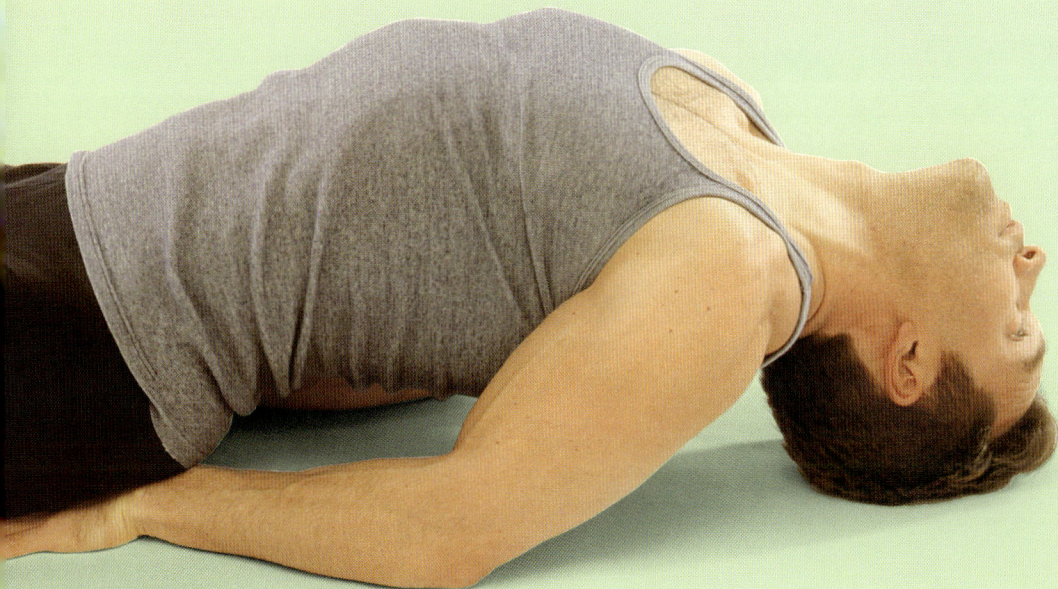

pascimottonasan

Forward bend posture

1 Sit with your legs outstretched and with your back and head erect but relaxed.

2 Breathe in as you raise your arms over your head and stretch your spine, lengthening it as much as possible.

3 Breathe out. Bending from the hips and not from the waist, stretch forward and grab your feet, ankles, or legs with your hands. (If necessary, wind a strap around your feet to assist in achieving this position).

4 Try to keep the back flat rather than rounded, even if it means your head does not go down as far. This is a stretch of the hamstrings (large muscles at the back of the thigh), as well as of the spine.

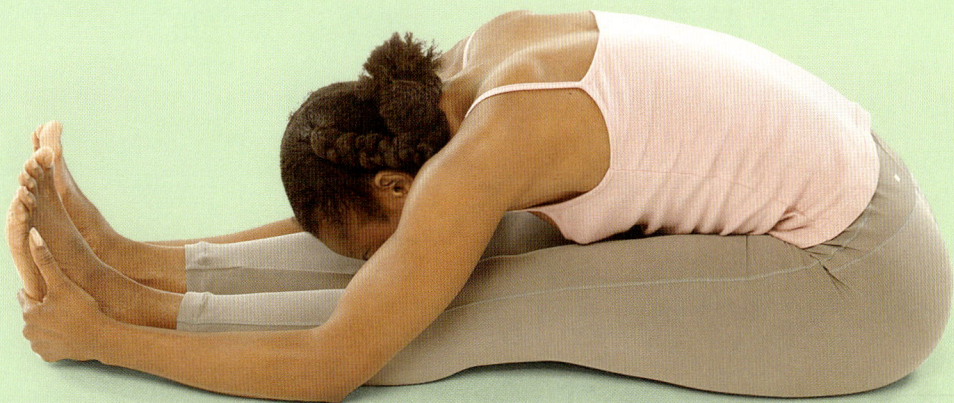

M

MEDIUM POSTURE

ustrasana—Camel posture

1 Kneel on the floor, holding your knees and feet together, and keeping your head and torso held erect. Place your hands on your hips and breathe in.

2 Holding your hips and thighs upright, breathe out, lean back, and place your hands on your heels. If you find it comfortable, allow your head to drop.

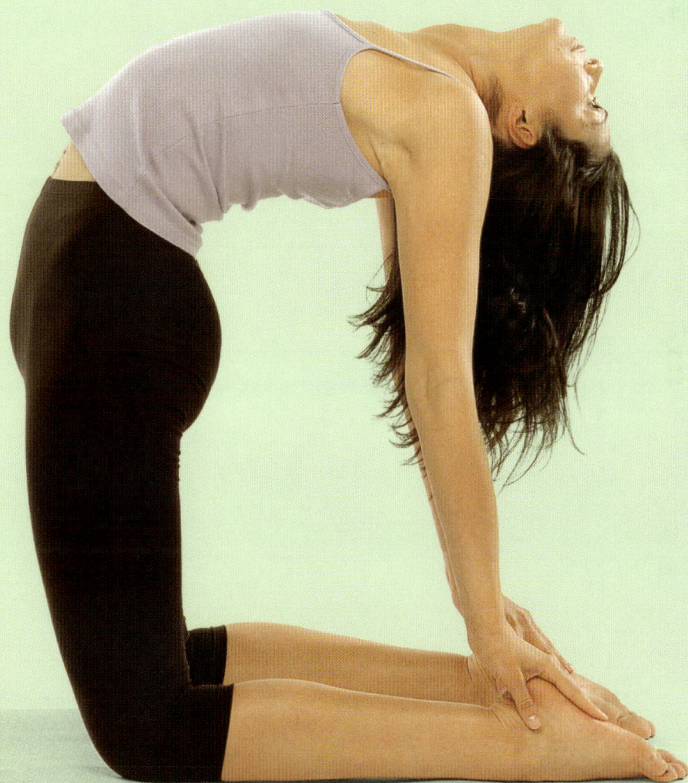

M

MEDIUM POSTURE

dhanurasana—Bow posture

1 Lie on your stomach with your forehead on the floor. Reach back with your hands and grasp your ankles.

2 Breathe in and lift your thighs, head, and torso off the floor. Look up in order to keep your chest raised.

3 Once you are in position, you can try to rock gently backward and forward to massage your internal organs.

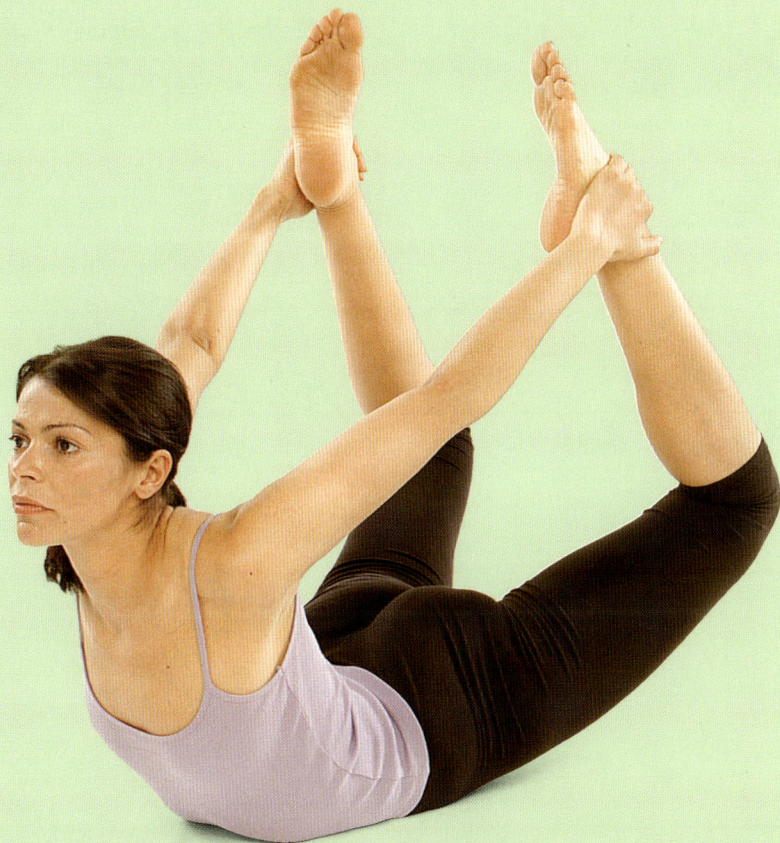

D

DIFFICULT POSTURE

chakrasana—Wheel posture

1 Lie on your back with your knees bent, feet close in to your buttocks, with your arms flat on the ground pointing toward your feet, hands palms down, or if they can reach comfortably, holding on to your ankles. Breathe in and lift your hips, keeping your head and shoulders on the ground.

2 If this position is comfortable and stable, place your hands behind your shoulders, palms downward, fingers pointing toward you. Breathe out.

3 Breathe in as you push yourself up on your hands and drop your head. Extend your legs as much as possible, keeping your feet on the floor and parallel with each other.

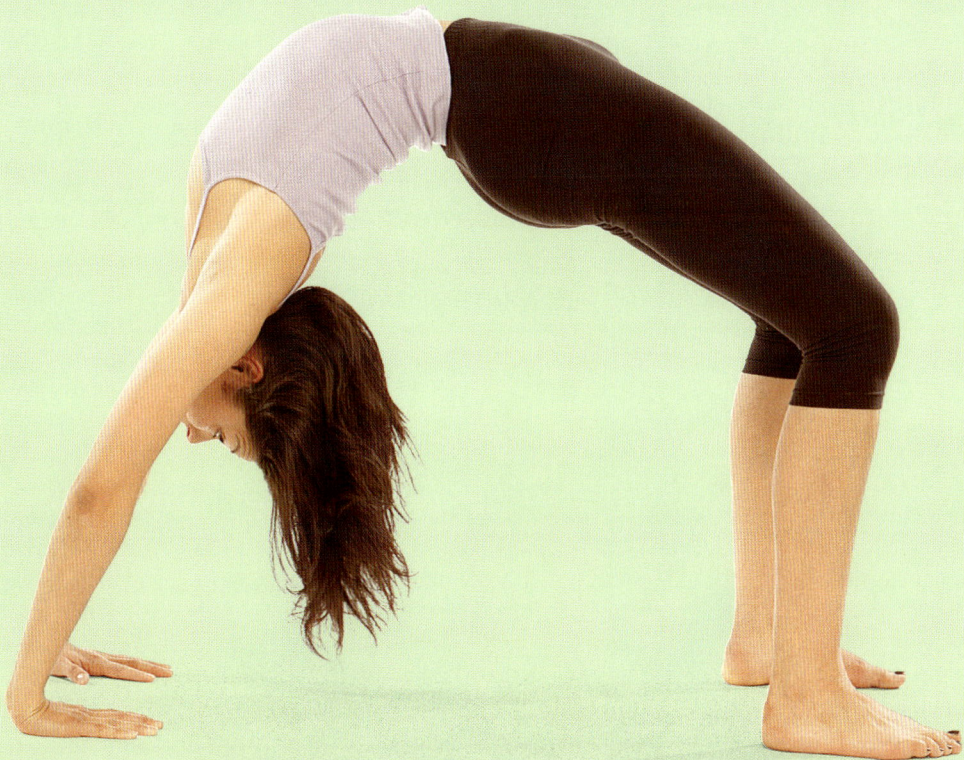

Yoga and flexibility

Yoga has long been recognized as one of the best forms of exercise to develop flexibility. The stretching exercises and movements performed by gymnasts and dancers are often modified yoga asanas. Although flexibility is one of the three components of physical fitness (along with strength and stamina), it is the most neglected in Western fitness culture. In the long run, flexibility serves us better than the ability to lift weights or run marathons.

To explain why yoga is so effective at developing flexibility, we need to consider the stretching mechanism itself. Flexibility is achieved by the stretching of the muscle fibers and associated connective tissues. When a muscle is contracted (made to work), the muscle fibers within it pull together causing it to shorten. Hence you see the bulge of the biceps when you bend your arm at the elbow and tense the muscle. When the biceps is in full contraction, it is not possible to move the elbow joint. When you relax the biceps again, it lengthens, and you can move your elbow freely.

Improvements in flexibility are in part due to the physical stretching of tissues, but also to our ability to relax a muscle at will. There are a further two physiological limitations on stretching: the stretch reflex, which contracts a muscle that is being stretched too much or too suddenly, and the Golgi tendon organs—a second safety device built into the tendons that link the muscles to bones, which inhibits contraction when a muscle either contracts or stretches too much. Both these safety mechanisms can be overcome by stretching slowly, and holding the stretch for at least fifteen seconds.

Yoga meets these two requirements perfectly, as the asanas require stretches to be held for extended periods, and also to stretch slowly. This de-activates both the stretch reflex and Golgi tendon organs. In addition, yoga uses the breath to increase the stretch, a technique also employed by athletes. Slowing and deepening the breath relaxes overall muscular tension, and stretching on the out-breath increases the joint's range of motion.

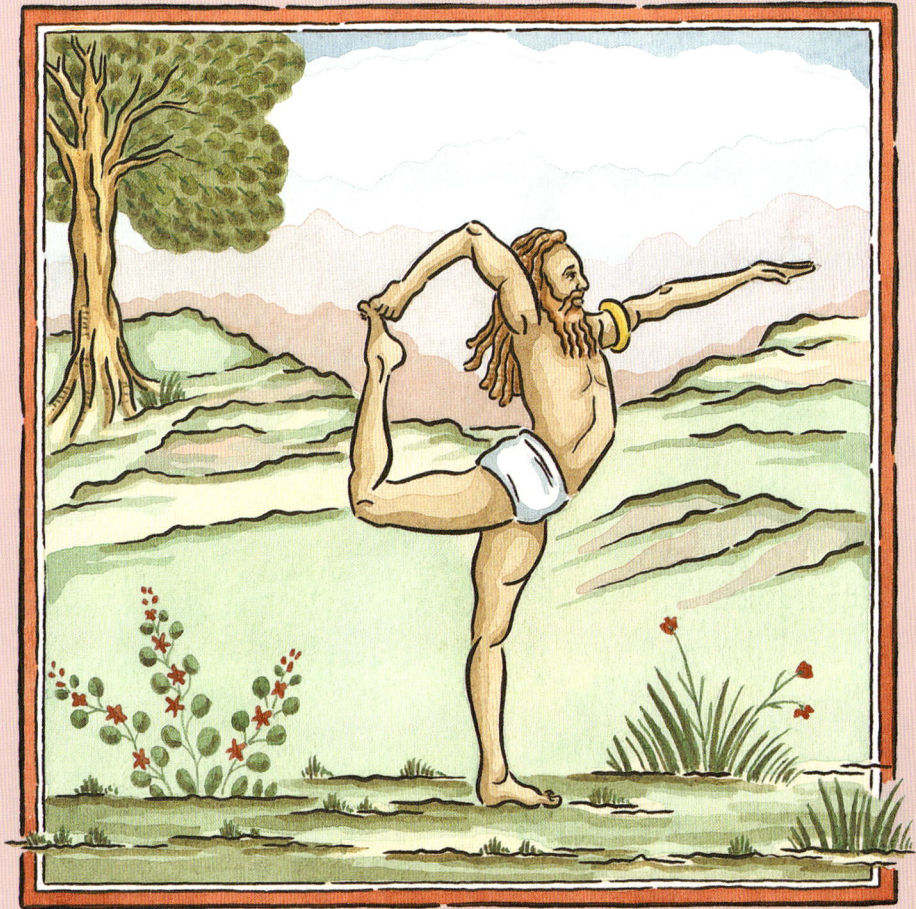

No pain, no gain?

This famous motto has haunted exercisers ever since it appeared in Jane Fonda's aerobics videos. How much should it hurt? In flexibility training, for some authorities, any pain, no matter how small, is a sign that the body is getting into trouble and that the stretch should be discontinued. Others encourage one to work through the pain barrier. The problem is that sensation is a totally subjective phenomenon, and so it is impossible for anyone to experience and evaluate what another person describes as painful, and we have to decide, from our own experience how much discomfort we should put ourselves through.

When I was in my twenties, I became very interested in stretching as a complimentary exercise to improve my performance in other sports and fitness activities. I set myself certain targets, such as achieving the box, or front splits within two years, and I employed stretching methods that would seem extreme to a student of yoga. In one technique, my stretching partner rested her full weight on my hips and buttocks as I lay on my stomach with my legs spread wide apart in a front split.

After a year of this kind of stretching, I was very close to achieving my goal. My stretching partners and I had quickly made the link between stretching and deep breathing, but we also noticed an unexpected release of emotional tension. After intense (and painful) sessions we would might feel saddened, sometimes to the point of tears, or at other times elated. It was as if the stretching was providing a physical outlet for unearthing buried memories and feelings.

When I later read about bodywork techniques such as Rolfing, which aim at relieving mental tension through physical manipulation, I realized that we had recognized an important, yet often misunderstood, aspect of the mind-body link.

It became quite clear to me that there is a physical aspect to experience and memory, and that we had learned how to release it by stretching.

Now in my forties, I would not put myself through the same agonizing procedures, nor recommend them to anyone else. I have, however, continued in my daily practice of stretching, in the past few years, returning to the formal study of Hatha yoga, as a mechanism to achieve that lightness of body and mind that I experience after a particularly good workout.

Siddhis: Miraculous powers

The siddhis are supernatural powers that can be attained when one is advanced in the practice of yoga. In the *Yoga Sutra*, Patanjali cites knowledge of the past and future, the power to make oneself invisible and leave one's body, and telepathy among the siddhis, but he warns the yogi that they can become obstacles to self-realization. Although some commentators of the *Yoga Sutra* believe in the literal reality of the siddhis, others argue that Patanjali's descriptions are not meant to be taken literally, but are symbolic of the spiritual attainments of the yogi.

It is thought that there are twenty three siddhis in all, and these have been graded into three classes; great, medium and small. While the "great" siddhis suggest supernormal attainment, the underlying message to be derived from the siddhis may be the importance of character, behavior and attitude, and ascetic control over the mind. In short, the purification of the inner self which is at the heart of yoga practice and philisophy. The escalation of the subtle and astral bodies too, is important for the realization of siddhis.

In his book, *Autobiography of a Yogi*, Parahamansa Yogananda, who was a pioneer of yoga in the United States in the twentieth century, describes miraculous events from the life of his teachers. While these stories were probably devised to amaze the credulous, there are two "miraculous feats" that have been observed and studied by respected Western authorities. The first is "Tumo," the heating of the body at will, which is done through a combination of pranayama techniques and meditation. The second is "burial alive," in which a yogi slows his breathing and heart rate to such an extent that he appears to be clinically dead. He is then interred, and later dug up and "resuscitated" by his followers.

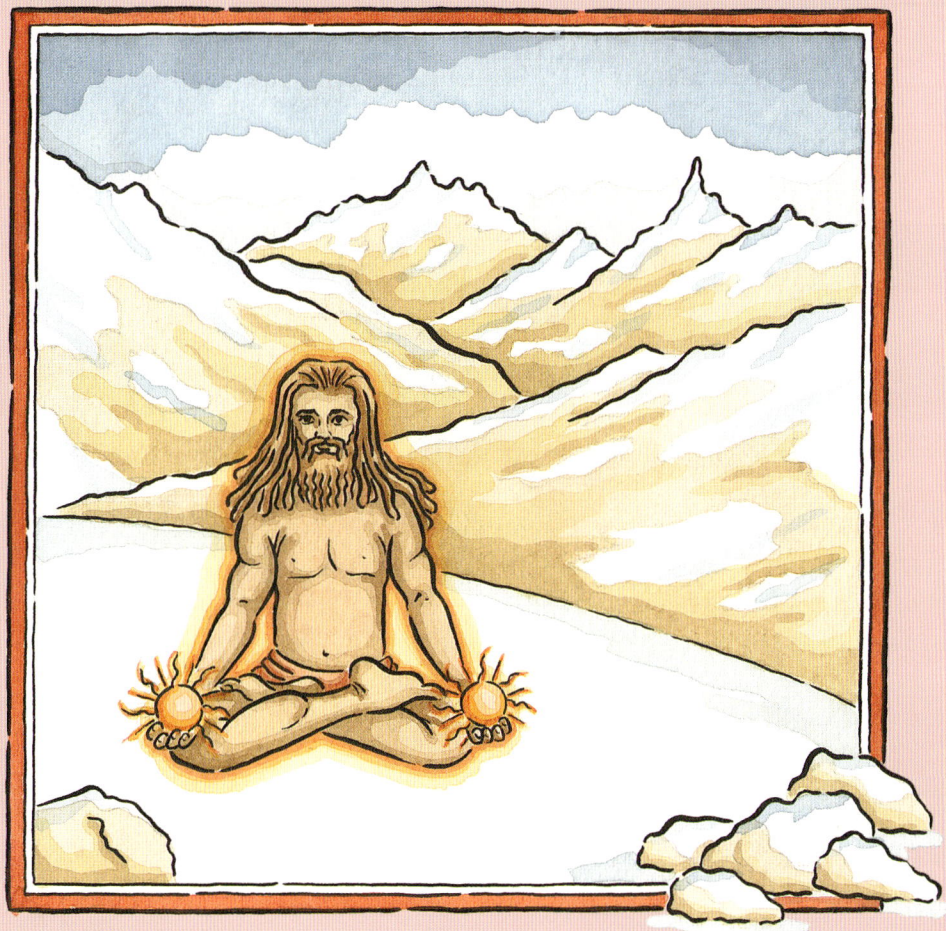

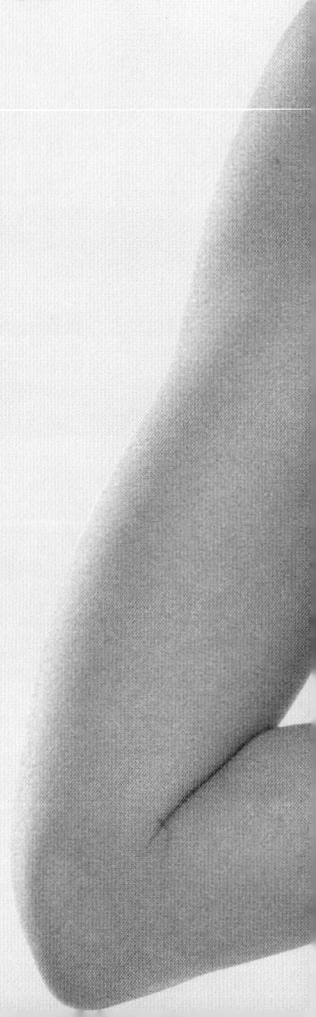

sarvangasana
invert

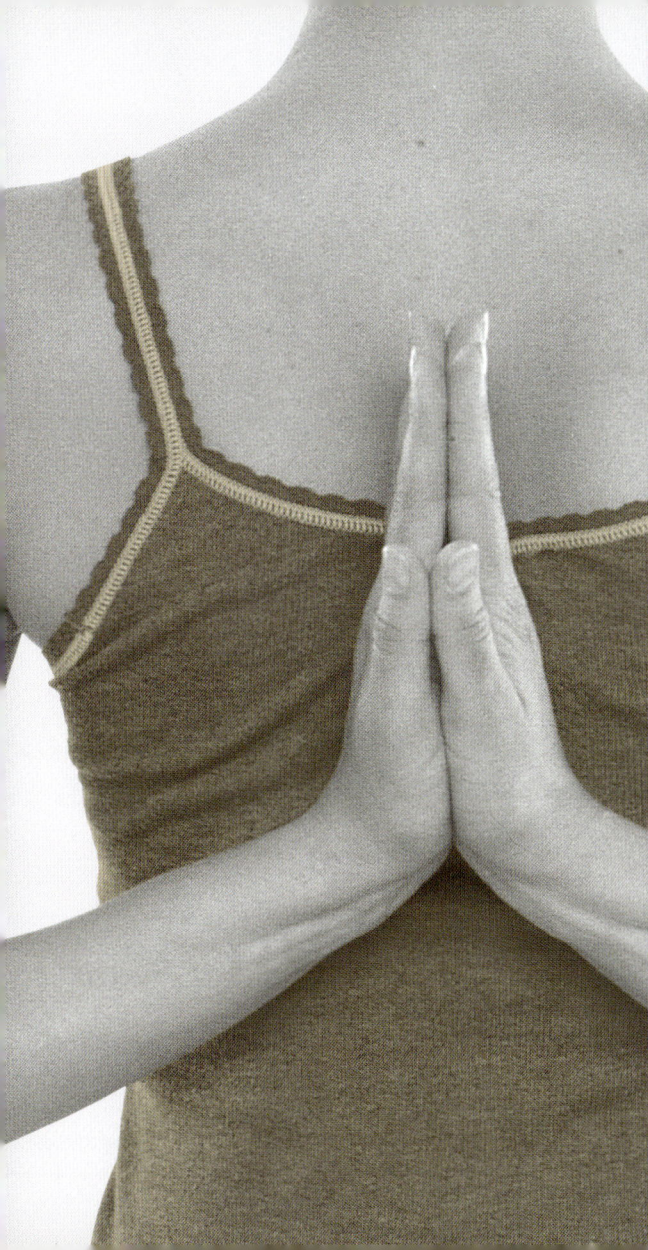

sarva means whole or
entire and *anga* means
body; so *Sarvangasana*
translates literally as
"whole-body pose."

chapter 6

benefits

It's probably true to say that very few of us have experienced the full inversion of our bodies since the days of childhood play. The physical postures of Hatha yoga challenge our most basic conceptions about how we stand, sit, and move—in this case it literally turns them on their head.

From a health point of view, the shoulder-stand is celebrated as one of the most beneficial of all asanas. In addition to curing flatulence and constipation, it is said to relieve tiredness in the morning, either if you have slept badly or overslept; and in the evening, to promote sleep. When the body is inverted, a supply of rich oxygenated blood bathes the organs and glands in the upper torso, including the brain, thyroid, and pituitary glands. The position of the head and neck is also said to regulate the functioning of the thyroid gland. In my own practice, I have found Sarvangasana particularly effective in curing headaches, and clearing a blocked nose.

"Work alone is your privilege, never the fruits thereof. Never let the fruits of action be your motive; and never cease to work."

Hatha Yoga Pradipika

inverted postures

In these postures, the inverted body is held on three different parts of the body—the shoulders, the head, or the arms and hands. In Sarvangasana, the shoulder-stand, and Halasana, the plough, the body is held on the shoulders. In Sirshasana, the headstand, the body is held by the head, and in Vrichikasana, the scorpion, and the Western gymnast's handstand (which is also an asana, though not included here), it is held by the arms and hands. In addition to the benefits of Sarvangasana already discussed, these asanas will develop overall balance, as well as strength and stamina in the arm and abdominal muscles.

Most averagely fit people should be able to perform Sirshasana, the headstand, if not at first attempt, then after a little practice. The reasons why people do not succeed are psychological rather than physical. First, there is the fear of falling and injuring oneself, and then the belief that it is just too difficult. Achieving (and holding) these postures helps one to develop courage and self-confidence.

Halasana, the plough, combines the benefits of the inverted asanas with those of the bending asanas, often helping to ease upper and lower back conditions. The contraction of the body during this asana also stimulates the digestive system and the thyroid gland.

"He who practises Sirshasana for three hours every day will conquer time."

Yoga Tatwa Upanishad

M

sarvangasana

Shoulder–stand posture

1 Lie on the floor with your legs outstretched, feet together, and your arms by your side, palms facing down. Breathe out. Breathe in, keeping your hips on the floor, and bring your legs up vertically, holding your knees straight.

2 Breathe out and then take a deep breath in. Press down on your hands, and lift your torso off the floor, moving your hands to support your lower back, until your body is in a vertical position resting on your neck and shoulders.

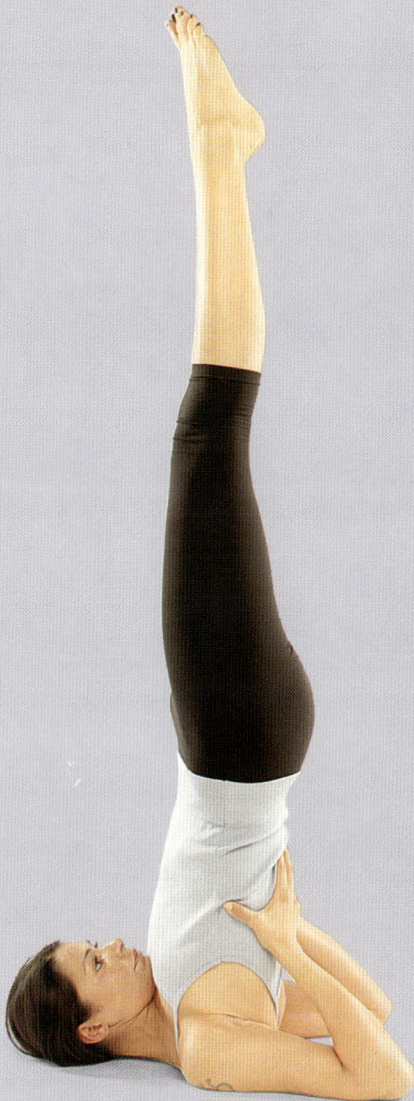

3 Your legs should be together and your knees held straight. Your chin is pressed into your chest. Do not turn your head in this position as you may injure your neck.

4 To return to the starting position, breathe out, bend your knees, and allow your legs to drop towards your head as you lower your torso, at first supporting yourself with your hands and then by pressing them into the floor. Do not allow yourself to drop suddenly but "unroll" your spine, vertebra by vertebra, until you are in Savasana.

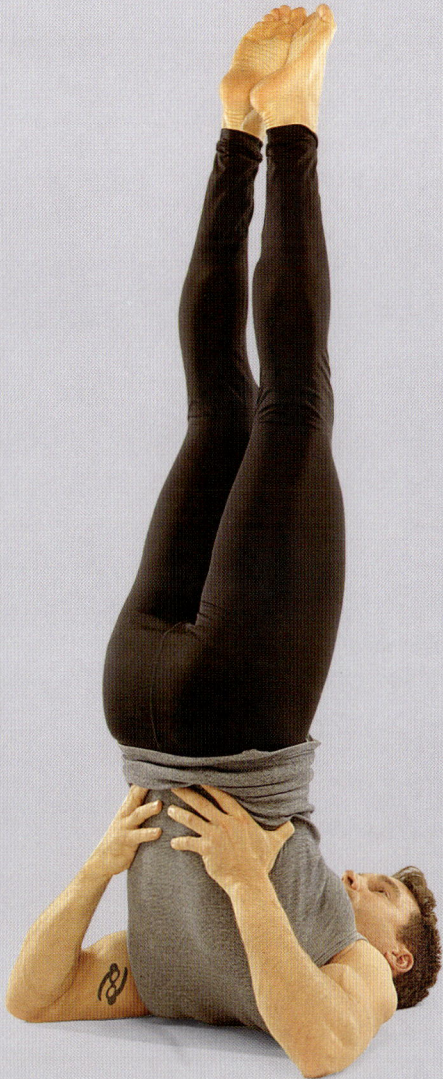

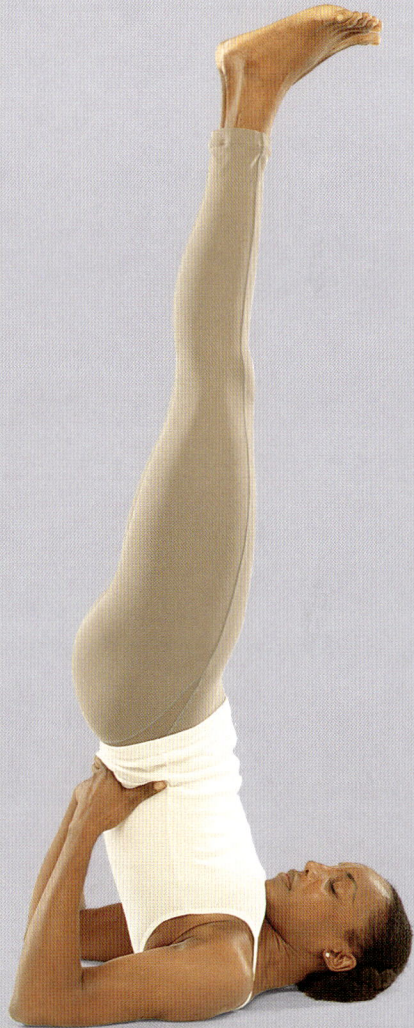

D

halasana—Plough posture

1 Lie on the floor with your legs outstretched, feet together, and your arms by your side, palms down. Breathe out. Breathe in, keeping your hips on the floor, and bring your legs up, keeping your knees bent.

2 Breathe out and in, press down on your hands, and lift your torso off the floor, moving your hands to support your lower back, until your body is resting on your neck and shoulders. Your legs, still bent at the knees, are now above your head.

3 Breathe out and straighten your legs, touching the floor with your toes directly behind the head if you can. Keep your feet together. (See opposite for variations in arm positions.)

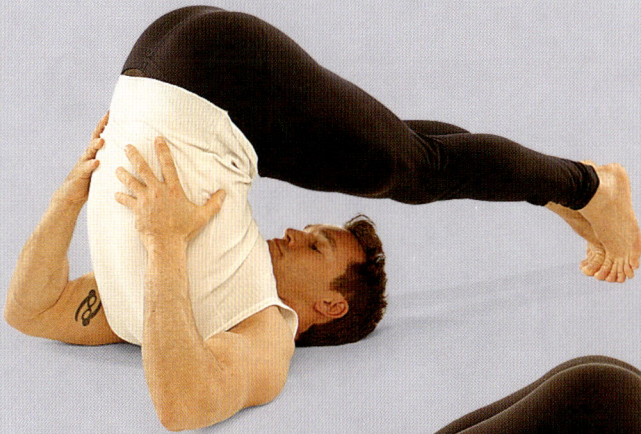

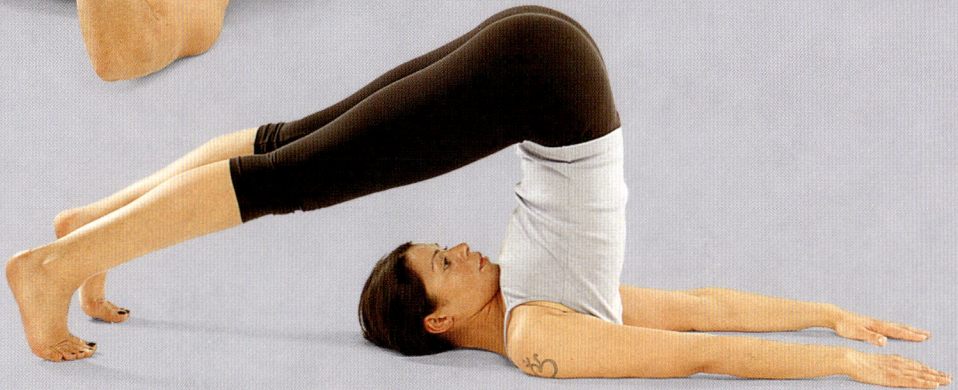

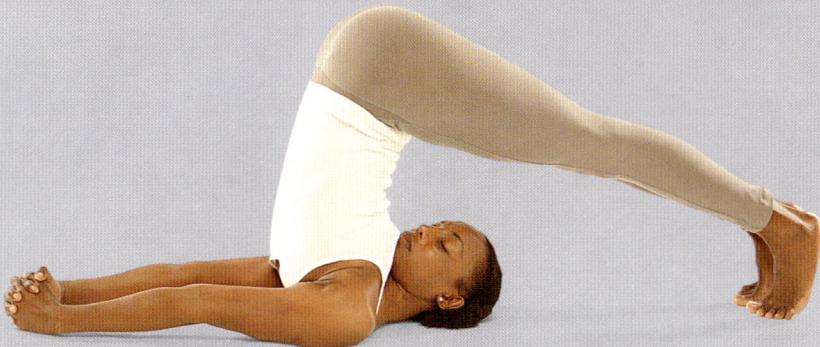

163

sirshasana—Headstand posture

1 Kneel and place your forearms on the floor in front while keeping the elbows shoulder-width apart. Interlace your fingers. Place the top of your head flat on the floor with the back of your head pressed against the inside of your interlaced fingers (figure 1).

2 Breathe in and stand onto your toes, and walk your feet toward your head (figure 2).

The sequence continues overleaf.

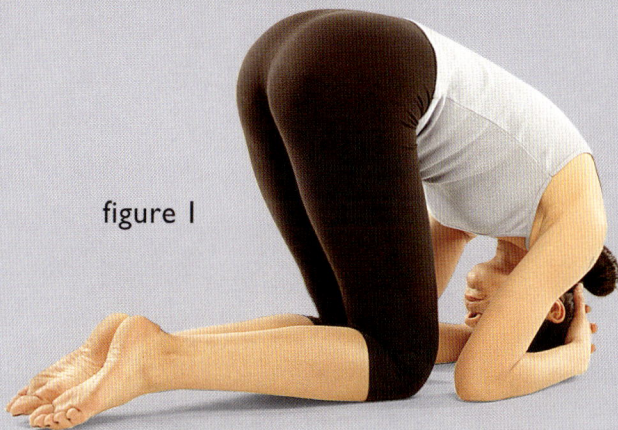

figure 1

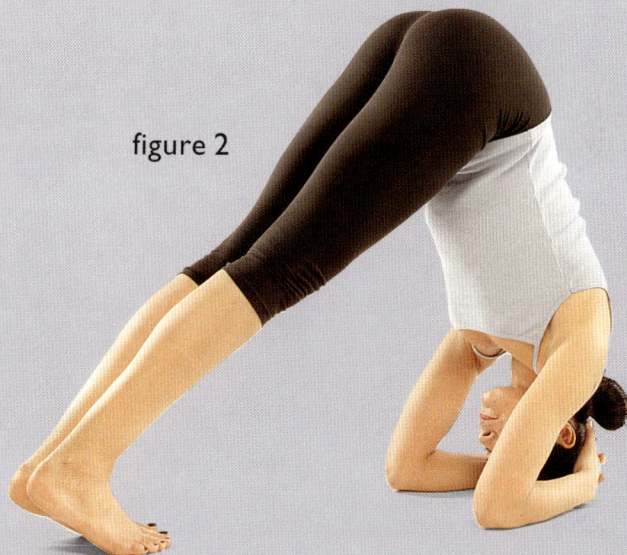

figure 2

3 Lift or kick your feet off the ground and raise your knees so that you are balanced on your head and forearms (figures 3 and 4).

4 Straighten your legs so that your body is balanced in a straight line (figure 5).

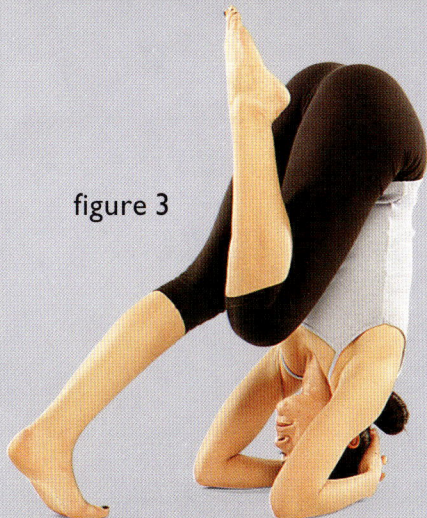

figure 3

figure 5

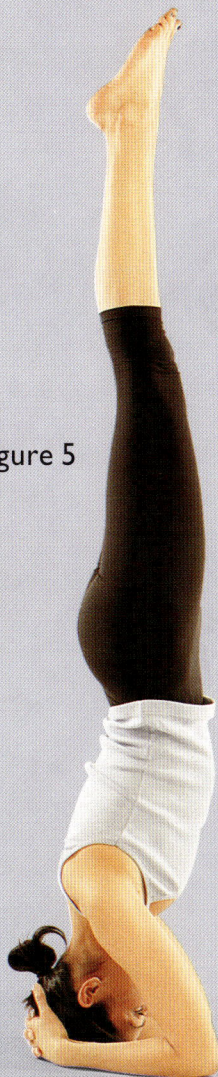

figure 4

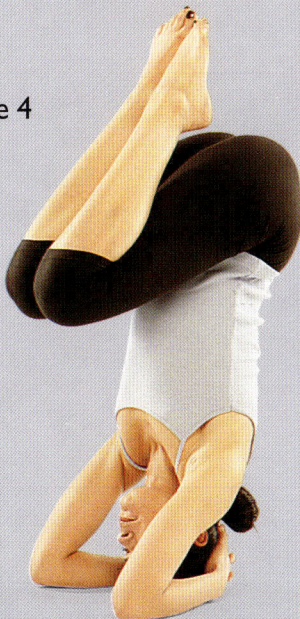

167

D

vrichikasana—Scorpion posture

1 Kneel on the floor and place your forearms flat on the floor, palms down, shoulder-width apart. Look forward, lifting your head as high as possible. Raise your buttocks and stand on your toes.

2 Breathe in and swing your legs up and over your head (figure 1). Slowly bend your knees and drop your feet toward your head. To avoid losing your balance, be careful not to move too quickly (figure 2).

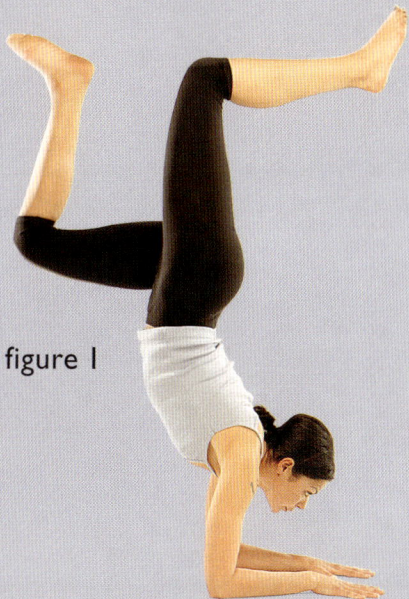

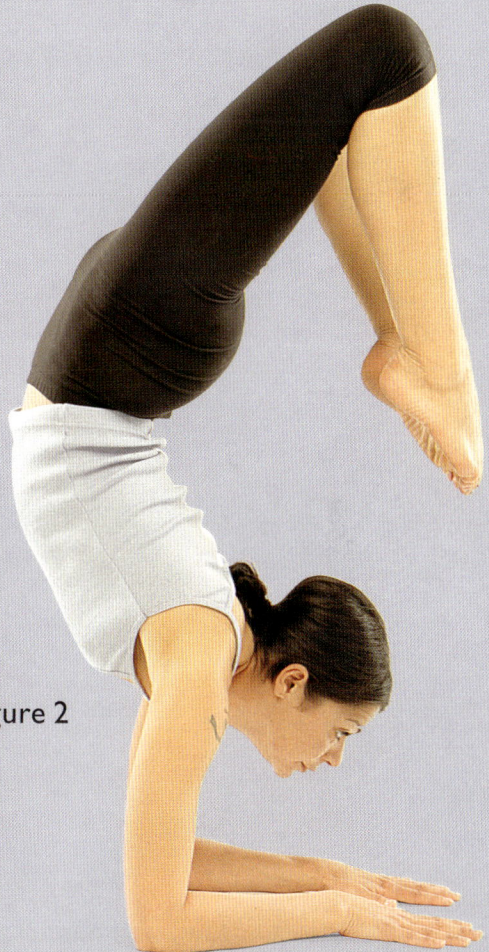

figure 1

figure 2

The Shariras: Understanding the three bodies

In the Hindu tradition, the Atman, or immortal true self or soul, is surrounded by three bodies, only one of which is visible to the human eye: the Sthula Sharira, the mortal body of flesh and bone. The two immortal bodies are the Suksma Sharira, the subtle or "astral" body, and the Karana Sharira, the body that can attain bliss, and which determines what your next incarnation will be. By following a correct diet and performing the asanas, the yogi brings the Sthula Sharira under his control. Through the performance of pranayama and meditation, the yogi attempts to transform his two immortal bodies and lead his Atman to attain Moksha, liberation from rebirth, and Samadhi, absorption into Brahman, the ultimate reality.

The Suksma Sharira:
The astral body

THE NADIS

The Suksma Sharira (also Linga Sharira) is composed of the seven chakras, or energy centers, and the nadis, the channels through which the prana flows to regulate the body's functions. There are said to be 72,000 main nadis, and many more secondary nadis. The principal nadi is the Sushumna which rises from the base of the spine to the top of the head, passing through the seven chakras. This central channel, which acts as the astral body's "spinal cord," is used during meditation. It is also the conduit of Kundalini (spiritual energy, see pages 210–13), that is released during Tantric practices. Intertwined around the Sushumna are the Pingala and Ida nadis, which are the main conduits of prana during our daily activities.

171

The Chakras

The chakras, which when translated means "wheels," are energy centers spaced along the Sushumna nadi at the points in the astral body where the nadis meet. Each is represented by a color, geometrical shape, number of lotus petals, and mantra (sound). Although there is no scientific evidence for the existence of the chakras and nadis, some authorities claim that there is a degree of concordance between their location in the astral body, and that of the major nerves and glands in the physical body. In visualization techniques, yogis consciously direct the flow of prana to certain chakras. The lower chakras are concerned with the physical plane of existence, while the higher chakras are gateways to the higher realms of the spirit.

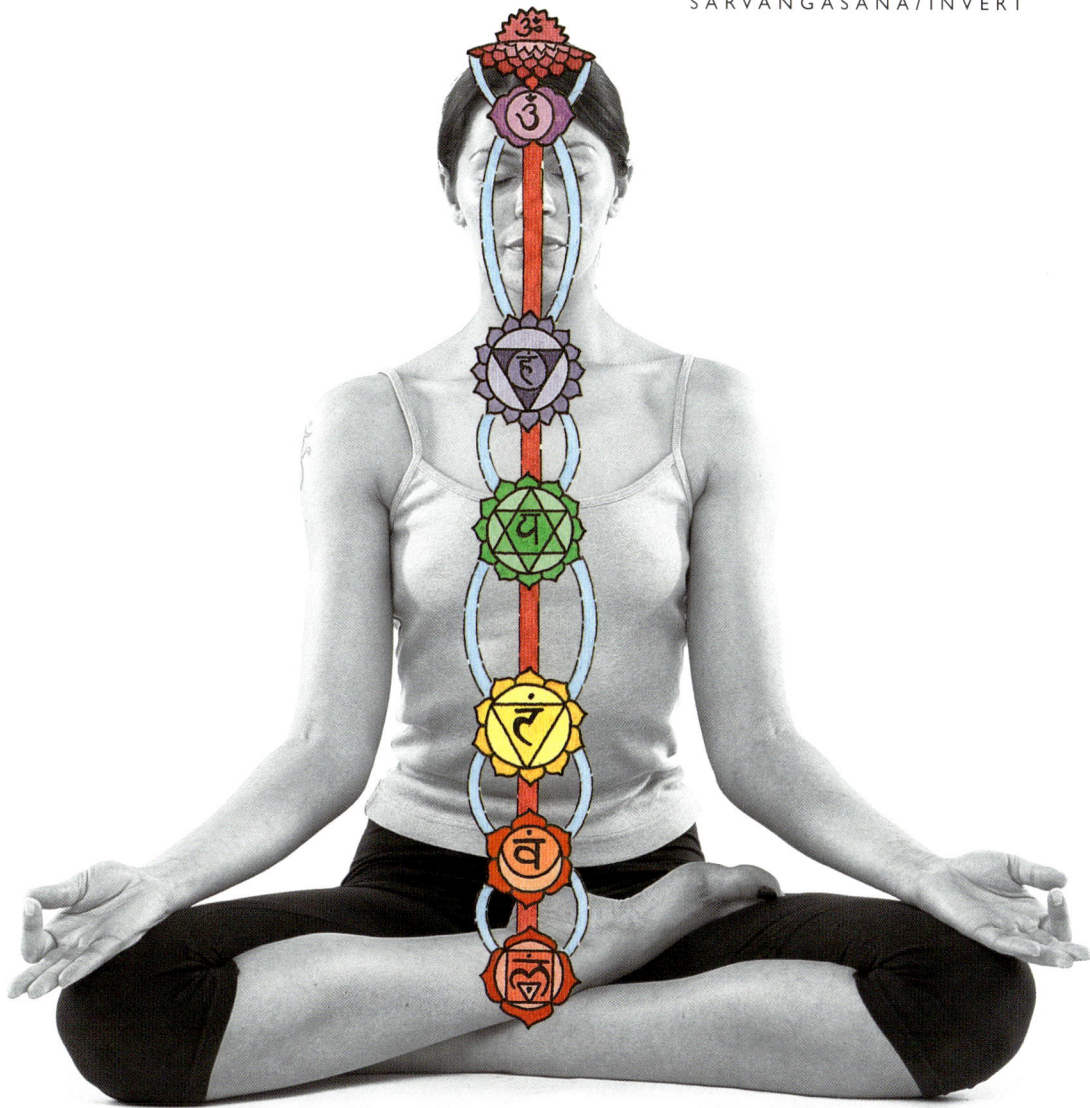

muladhara chakra

root

COLOR: RED

ELEMENT: EARTH

MANTRA: LAM

NUMBER OF PETALS: FOUR

TUTELARY GOD AND GODDESS: BRAHMA AND DAKINI

Located at the base of spine between the anus and the sexual organs, Muladhara is the closest chakra to the earth and represents earthly grounding. It governs the physical body, including the sensations of pain, sensuality, pleasure, and power, and also our drive to survive. It is associated with the adrenal glands and the kidneys. It is also believed to be the location of Kundalini, the body's spiritual energy (see pages 210–13).

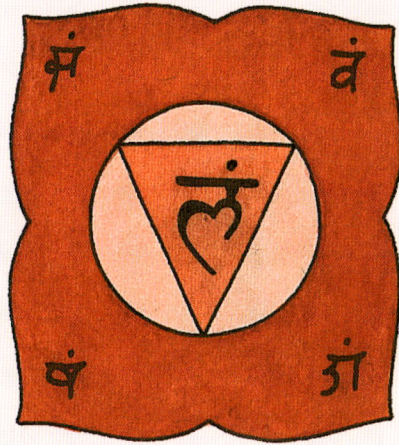

swadhishtana chakra

pelvic

COLOR: ORANGE

ELEMENT: WATER

MANTRA: VAM

NUMBER OF PETALS: SIX

TUTELARY GOD AND GODDESS: VISHNU AND RAKINI

Located at the sexual organs, Swadhishtana chakra represents sexuality, creativity, and the emotions of anger, resentment, and frustration. Governed by the element water, it relates to the sexual organs, as well as the liquid functions of the body: the circulation of the blood, urination, and sexual fluids.

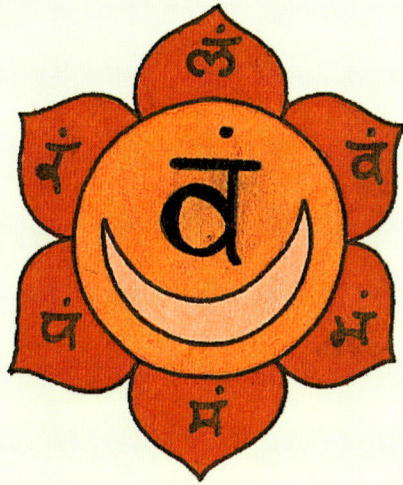

manipura chakra

solar plexus

COLOR: YELLOW

ELEMENT: FIRE

MANTRA: RAM

NUMBER OF PETALS: TEN

TUTELARY GOD AND GODDESS:
RUDRA AND LAKINI

Located in the solar plexus, a few inches above the navel, Manipura chakra is the seat of the emotions. It is also related to the mental or intellectual body, including thoughts, opinions, and judgments. Manipura governs the adrenal glands, pancreas, liver, stomach, and the nervous system.

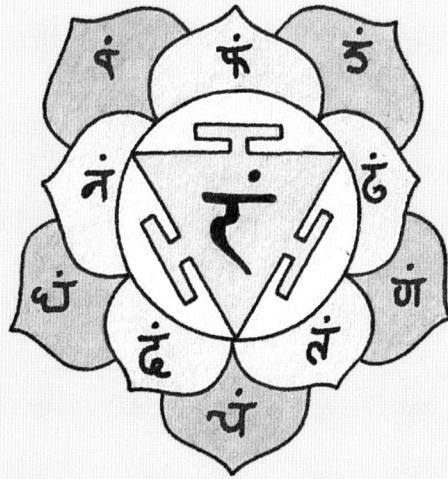

anahata chakra

heart

COLOR: GREEN

ELEMENT: AIR

MANTRA: YAM

NUMBER OF PETALS: TWELVE

TUTELARY GOD AND GODDESS: ISHA AND KAKINI

Located at the heart, Anahata is the chakra of love, harmony, and peace. We fall in love through Anahata chakra, from whence the emotion moves to Manipura chakra, and to the lower sexual chakra where it creates strong feelings of sexual attraction. Anahata is the first chakra to extend beyond the realm of earthly matter. It acts as the bridge between the realms of spirit and matter. It is associated with the circulation, and the immune system and endocrine systems.

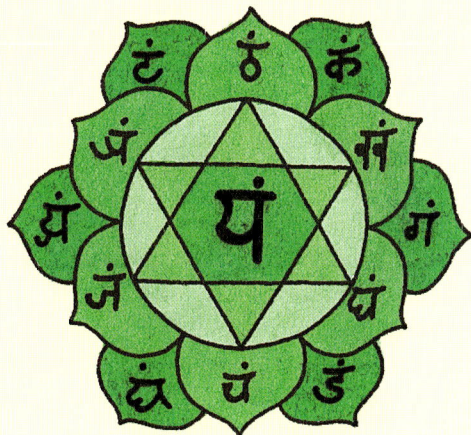

vishuddha chakra

throat

COLOR: BLUE

ELEMENT: SOUND

MANTRA: HAM

NUMBER OF PETALS: SIXTEEN

TUTELARY:
SADASHIVA AND SAKINI

Located within the throat, Visuddha is the chakra of communication, expression, and judgment. If you have problems of the throat, imagine that your throat is bathed in a blue light. Visuddha governs the thyroid and parathyroid glands, lungs, vocal cords, and bronchial apparatus.

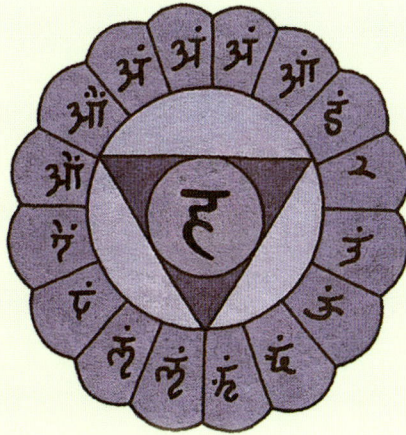

ajna chakra

third eye

COLOR: INDIGO

ELEMENT: LIGHT

MANTRA: OM

NUMBER OF PETALS: TWO

TUTELARY GODDESS: HAKINI

Located in the middle of the forehead, Ajna chakra, the "third eye," is thought to be the seat of our inner vision, dreams, gifts of clairvoyance, wisdom, and perception. We use this chakra for visualization, receiving insight or inspiration. It is associated with either the pineal or pituitary glands.

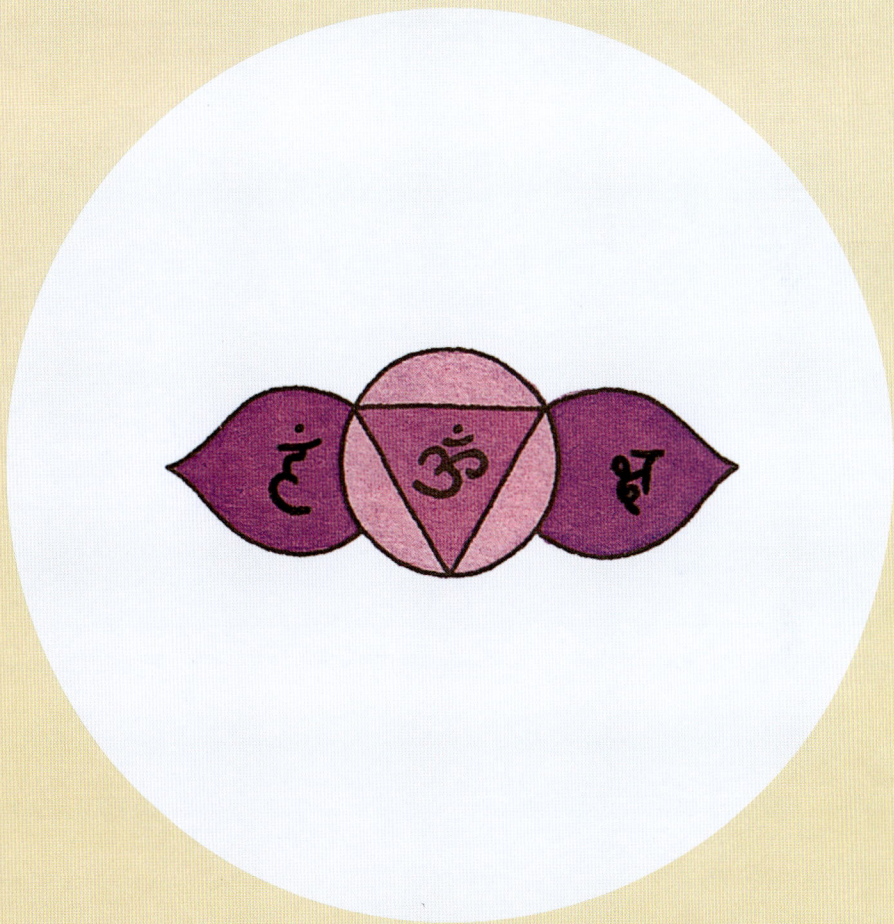

sahasrara chakra

crown

COLOR: WHITE

ELEMENT: THOUGHT

NUMBER OF PETALS: INFINITE

TUTELARY GOD: SHIVA

Located at the top of your head, Sahasrara is the chakra of divine purpose and destiny. It balances the interior and the exterior, and brings them into a harmonious whole. This chakra is said to be your own place of connection to God. It represents our belief systems, both conscious and unconscious. According to the same traditions, this chakra also governs the pituitary or pineal glands.

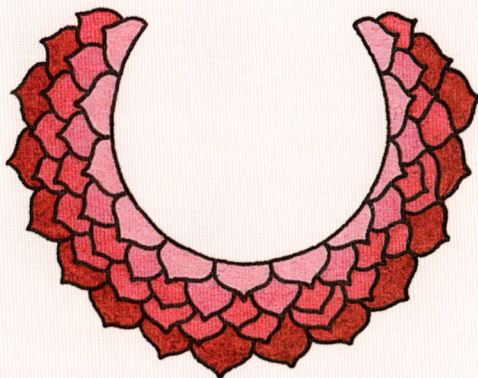

Ayurveda: Science of life

Ayurveda, which means "the science of life," is one of the oldest medical traditions in the world, dating back to India's Vedic period in the second millennium B.C.E. For many centuries, it was also the world's most advanced medical system. Ayurvedic doctors were the first to recognise the circulation of blood (during the eighth century B.C.E.), and employed smallpox vaccination centuries before Edward Jenner introduced it to Britain in the eighteenth century.

In Ayurveda the human body is governed by three basic principles, or doshas: vata, pitta, and kapha. Although we are subject to fluctuating patterns of the three doshas during the day, each individual has a unique combination of doshas, determined by the doshas of his or her parents at the moment of conception. Personality, body type, and intellectual capacities are determined by the dominance of one or more dosha. For example, a predominantly kapha dosha person is said to be heavily built, slow, and strong, while a vata type is either tall and strongly built or small and slight. The differences also extend to the mental sphere, and to the kinds of disease to which the individual may be susceptible.

Ayurvedic medical traditions developed long before the discovery of bacteria and viruses, so these play no part in the Ayurvedic theory of disease. The main cause of disease are instead imbalances in the three doshas, and improper diet and lifestyle, and the accumulation of toxins in the body. In response to a diagnosis, an Ayurvedic practitioner will prescibe herbal treatments, along with diet and exercise programs. These may include asanas and pranayama, as well as detoxifying therapies, such as aromatherapy and oil massages, and Vasti, colonic irrigation.

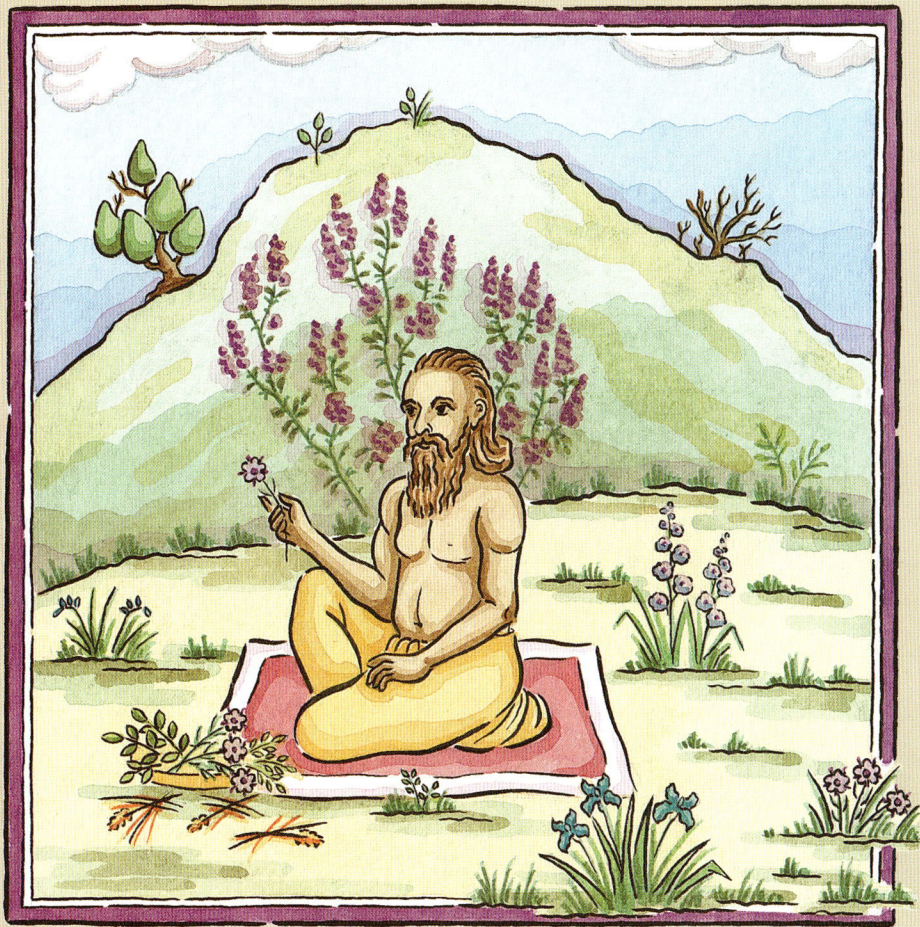

ardha—
matsyendrasana
twist

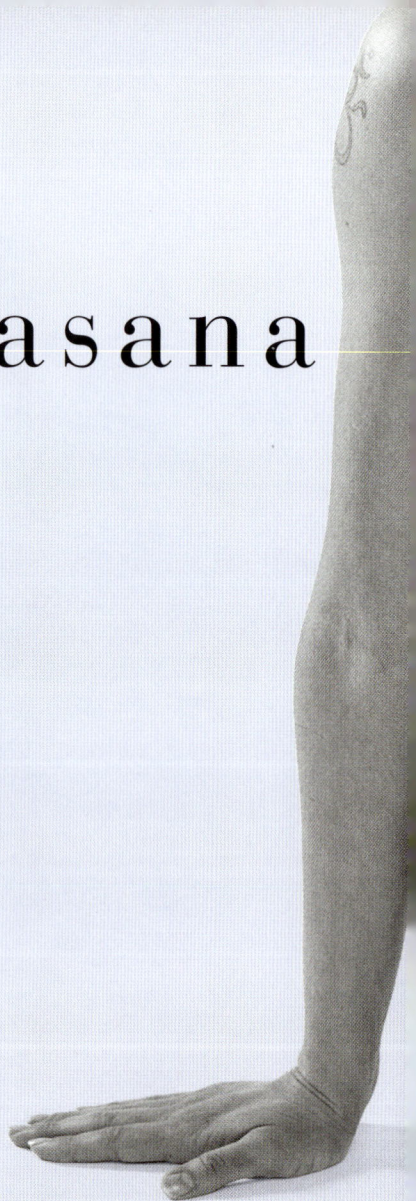

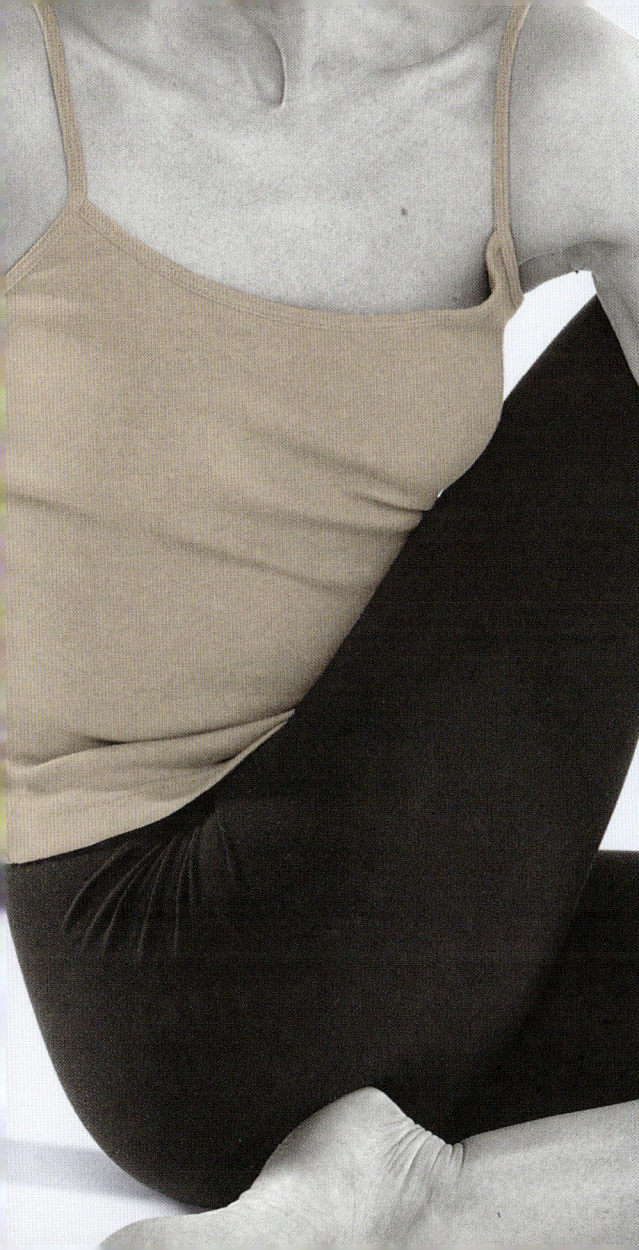

Matsyendra is one of the legendary founders of yoga, and this asana is dedicated to him. Ardha, meaning half, indicates that this is an easier version of the full posture.

chapter 7

benefits

The half-spinal twist, Ardha-Matsyendrasana, and the more challenging Matsyendrasana, the full spinal twist (see pages 204–5), are among of the most effective asanas in developing the rotational flexibility of the trunk. The alternating compression and release of the abdominal region improves the circulation and massages the internal organs, relieving digestive problems, as well as toning up the abdominal, lower back, and hip muscles. In combination with the bending asanas (see pages 126–45), they will counteract the stiffness caused by stress, poor posture, or prolonged periods of sitting in one position (at a computer, for example).

In esoteric schools of yoga, Ardha-Matsyendrasana is one of the asanas used to rouse Kundalini, the body's latent spiritual energy that is coiled around the base of the spine (see p210–13).

twisting postures

The spine is the largest joint in the body. A complex structure, it is composed of twenty-six vertebrae connected by tough intervertebral discs made of cartilage that act as shock absorbers. The bending asanas stretch the spine in its forward and backward flexion, but these asanas provide an opportunity for the spine to be exercised in rotation. There are few movements in daily life or in conventional exercise that allow for the spine to be stretched in this way.

The following asanas start with the easy Supine twist that can also be used as part of a warm-up program. The seated twists can also be performed while seated in a straight-back chair and using the back and arms of the chair to pull yourself around.

ardha–matsyendrasana

Half-spinal twist posture

1 Sit on the floor with your legs outstretched. Bend your right knee and place your right foot on the outside of your left knee.

2 Bend your left knee so that your left foot ends up next to your right buttock. If you need the support, place your right hand directly behind you. If not, hold it around your lower back.

3 Raise your left arm, stretching your spine, and bring it down so it rests on the right side of your right leg. Twist your spine and look over your right shoulder. Hold and repeat on the other side.

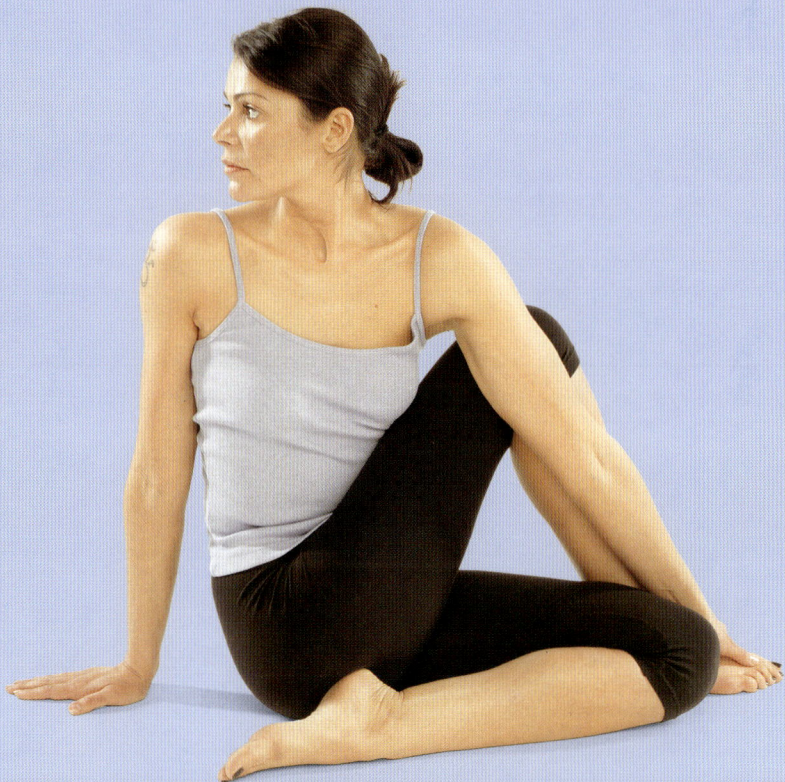

E

Supine twist

1 Lie on the ground with your legs outstretched. Breathe in as you bend your right knee and place your right foot on your left knee.

2 Breathe out and pull your right knee to the left until it touches the floor.

3 Turn your head to the left, twisting your spine while still keeping your shoulders on the ground. Hold and repeat on the other side.

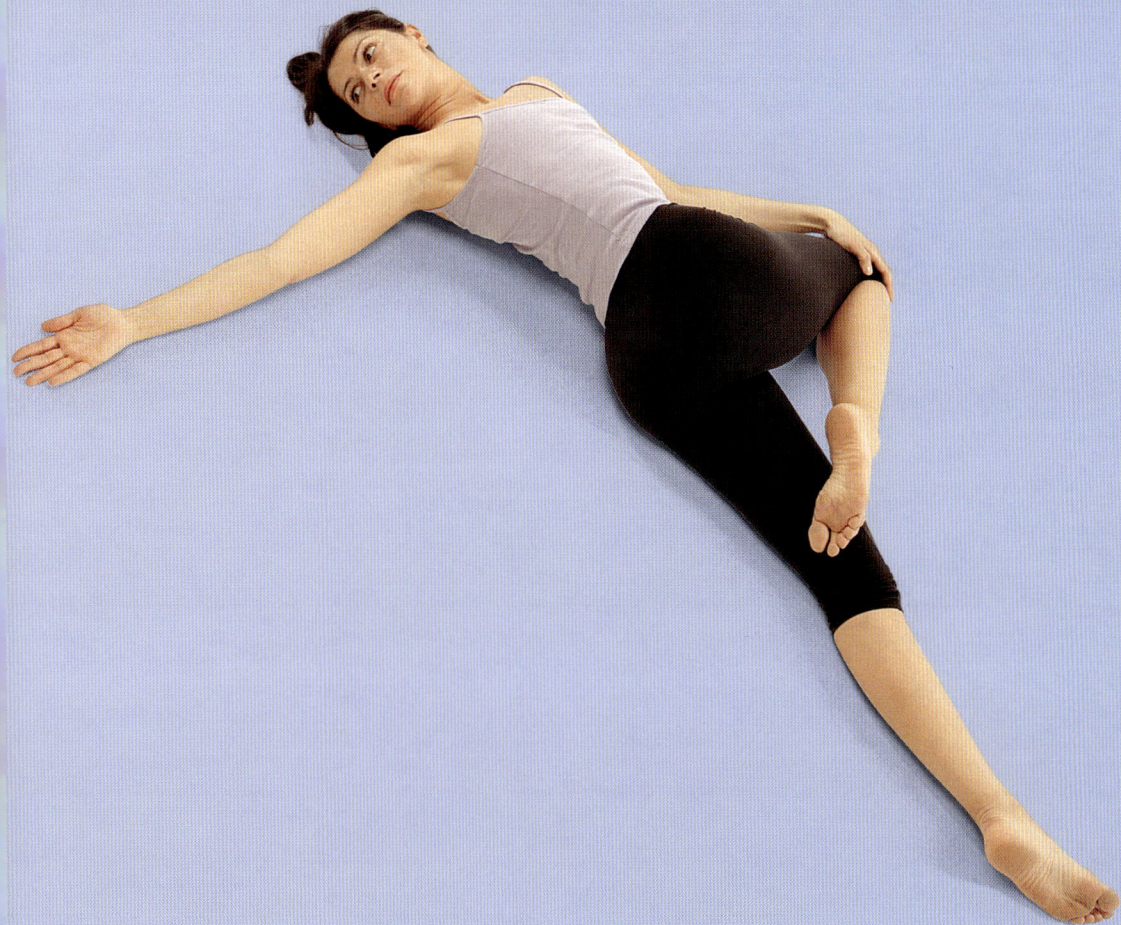

E

jatara parivartanasana

Turning the belly pose

I Lie on your back. Stretch your arms straight out to the side. Breathe out and raise your legs. Straighten the knees, so that your legs are perpendicular to your body.

2 Breathe out and lower your legs to the floor slowly and smoothly, without lifting the hips or your shoulders off the floor. Breathe in. Return the legs to the center, hold for a moment, and then lower to the other side.

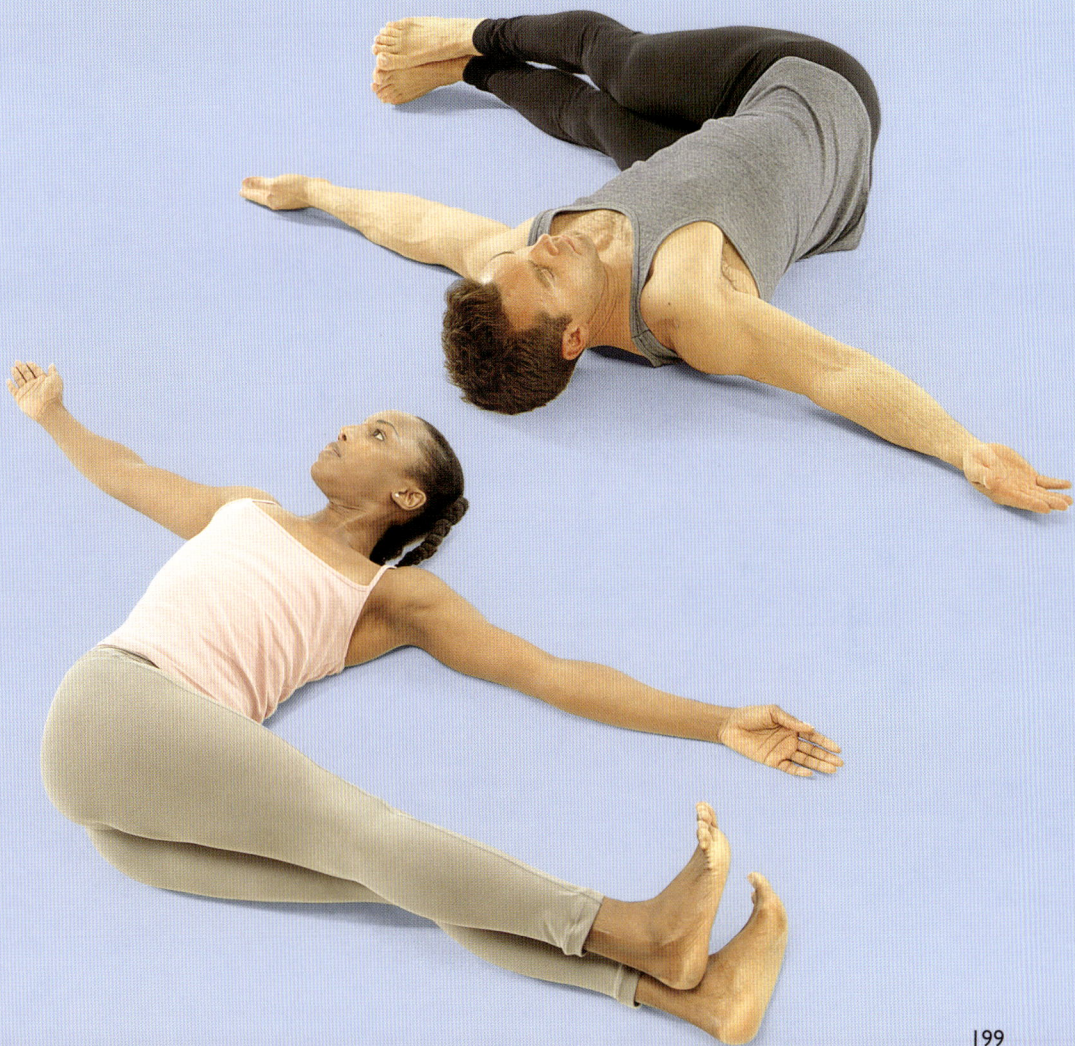

M

parivritta trikonasana

This standing twisting pose is often performed immediately after Trikonasana (see Standing poses, pages 82–93) of which it is a variation.

1 Stand in Tadasana. Jump or step about three feet apart. Breathe in and extend both arms to the side, keeping them parallel to the floor, palms facing down.

2 Breathe out and twist all the way around to place your right hand on the outside of your left foot. Turn your head and look up at your outstretched left hand, trying to align your shoulders, chest, and arms. Hold and repeat on the other side.

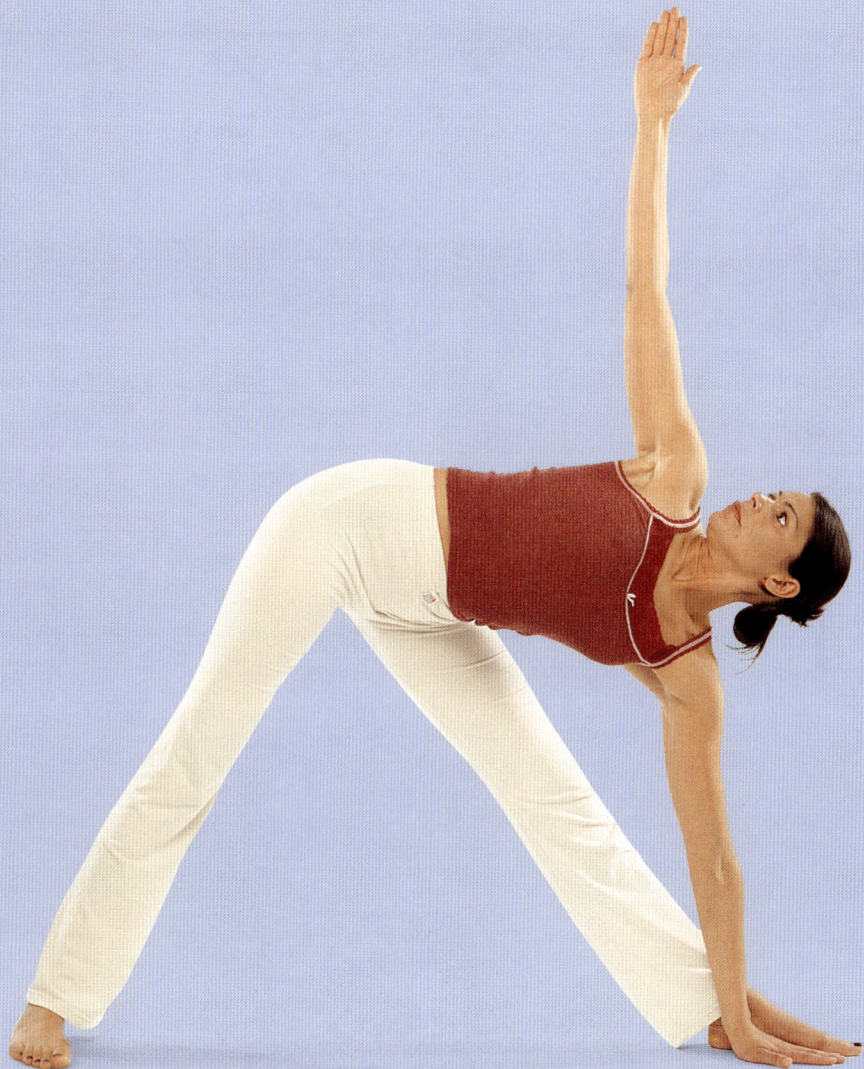

M

marichyasana—Marichi's posture

1 Sit on the floor with your legs outstretched in front of you. Breathe in as you bend your left knee, placing the left foot close in to your body but not touching your right thigh.

2 Breathe out, turn your body to the right as far as possible, and bring your left arm over your left thigh. Use your right arm for support. Pushing against your left arm and keeping your spine upright, continue to turn your body toward the right. Hold and repeat on the other side.

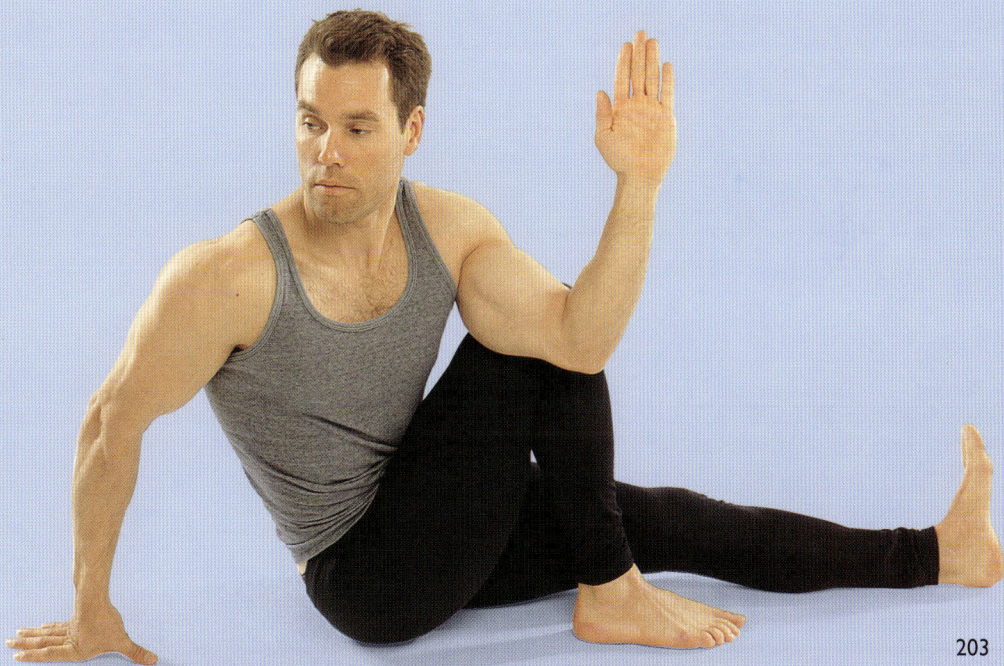

D

matsyendrasana—Full spinal twist

1 Sit on the floor with your legs extended in front of you. Breathe in, then bend your right knee and place your right foot high up on your left thigh, with the sole of your foot facing upward.

2 Bend your left knee and put your left foot next to the outside of your right knee. Reach your hands behind your back as shown if you can (or take hold of your left foot with your right hand), and look over your shoulder. Hold and repeat on the other side.

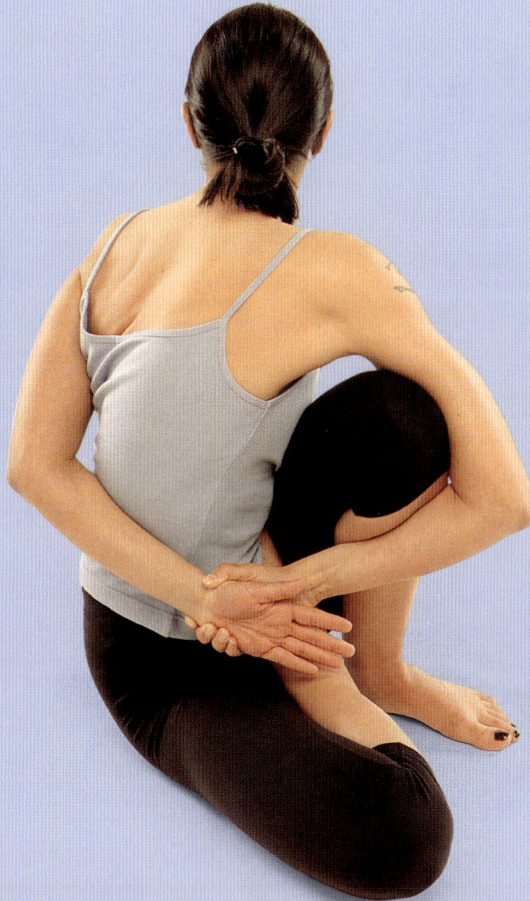

Yoga and sex

On the purely physical level, the practice of yoga will benefit your sex life by improving your general level of fitness, and in particular your flexibility and muscular endurance. The control of the breath taught by pranayama techniques will help to control excitement during intercourse, and the mental and physical relaxation that pranayama and meditation develop may make it a more intense experience.

In combination, these will help to tackle premature ejaculation, a common problem among men of any age, and facilitate orgasm for women. Several of the asanas, such as Bhujangasana and Dhanurasana, in the bending asanas (see pages 126–45), are recommended for sexual problems. There are also traditions in yoga, evident in ancient and modern practice (see page 206), that make use of sex for spiritual fulfillment.

Sex and sexual symbolism have always played an important role in Hindu religion. In a Freudian echo, the myth of Shiva's lingam (phallus) tells how the god's infinitely long sexual organ, once it had become detached from his body, threatened to destroy the Universe. The Universe was saved when the lingam was coupled with the yoni (vagina). In temples dedicated to Shiva, the god is symbolized by a representation of the lingam-yoni coupling. The sexual act itself has been sanctified in various ways in Hinduism, and until the modern period, several cults employed deva-dasis, or temple prostitutes.

Although chastity is one of the virtues followed by the yogi, we have seen that there are exceptions, such as the case of a partnered yogi. However, some unmarried yogis, who stand outside the caste system and have rejected the strict code of behavior expected of the Brahmin, exploit their powers and knowledge for sexual ends. The Rajneesh movement, in particular, was criticized for the alleged sexual excesses of its members.

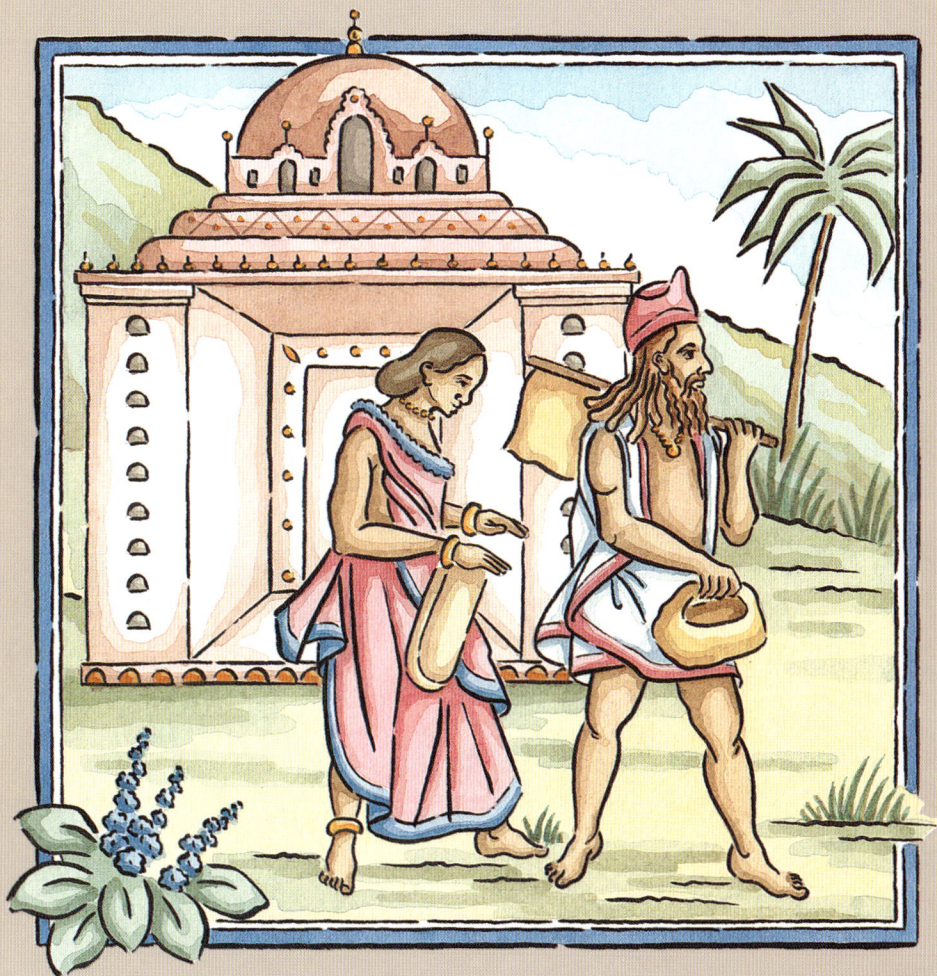

Tantra yoga

Tantra yoga, which is based on a set of fifth century sacred texts known as the Tantras, is a complex mixture of meditative practices and magical rituals intended to lead the Tantrika to Moksha and Samadhi.

Called the "Left Hand Path" by followers of more orthodox yogas because participants break Brahmanic law by eating forbidden foods, such as meat, drinking, and taking drugs, Tantra seeks to harness the power of sexuality to achieve spiritual ends. In the ritual of Maithuna, or sacred coitus, the participants represent the male and female principles, Shiva and Shakti, and also the Atman and Brahman.

The habitual secrecy of Tantric schools and the rumors surrounding their practices have made followers of other yogas suspicious and critical. When Westerners first encountered Tantra yoga in the nineteenth century, they were shocked by its overtly sexual nature. Today, attitudes to sexuality have changed to such an extent that the West is more open to Tantric knowledge.

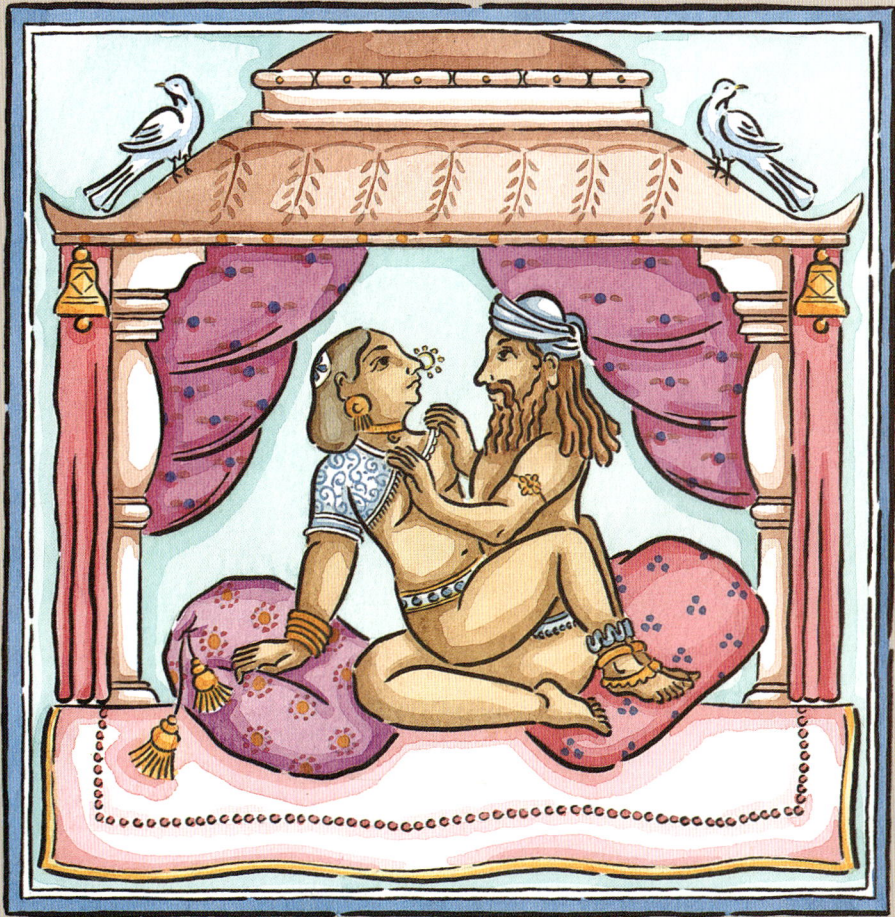

Kundalini: Spiritual energy

Kundalini is a form of spiritual energy that is represented as a snake coiled at the base of the Sushumna nadi, the central channel of the astral body (see page 71) in the Muladhara chakra (see pages 174–5). The release of Kundalini is believed to lead to Moksha, or liberation from the cycle of rebirth. Seen as the body's feminine energy, Kundalini is aroused through the use of asanas, pranayama techniques, mantras, and bandhas. Once aroused, Kundalini releases intense heat. It rises up the Shusumna, piercing the chakras, until it reaches the Sahasrara chakra (see pages 186–7) at the crown of the head, uniting the male and female polarities of the body. In some traditions, the Kundalini then descends, filling the body with the "nectar of bliss."

The practice is reported to be highly dangerous and very few gurus have ever claimed to have succeeded in raising Kundalini to the seventh chakra. A school specializing in teaching Kundalini yoga has been founded by Yogi Bhajan.

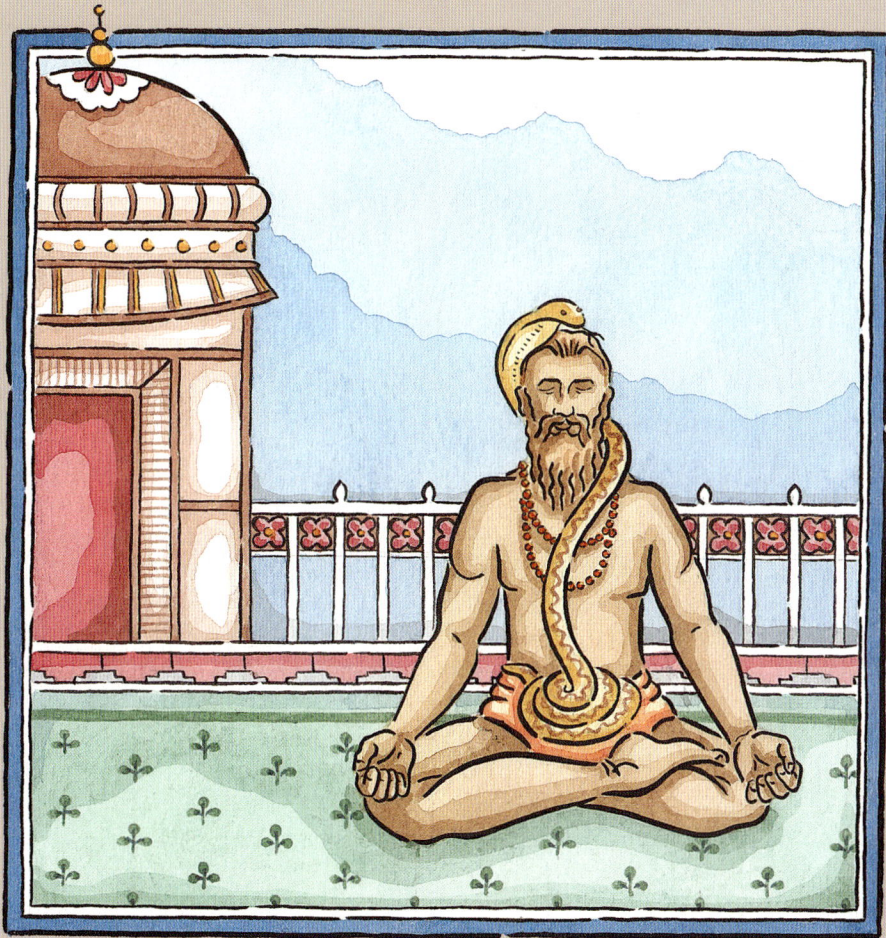

Retaining the life force

In certain traditions seminal fluid is seen as a substance charged with supernatural powers. Even in the scientifically advanced West, doctors once endorsed the Biblical prohibition against the "Sin of Onan," by warning that the masturbator would fall prey to physical and mental feebleness. One of my t'ai chi ch'uan teachers was the first (but not the last) to tell me that, "It takes one hundred mouthfuls of food to create one drop of blood, and one hundred drops of blood to create one drop of semen." The implication being that it was a criminal act to "waste" it. In Tantra yoga, semen is equated with the life force, and its retention is said to have the power to overcome death itself.

Withholding semen is a routine part of Tantric sexual practices, as ejaculation would interrupt the contemplative nature of Maithuna. Even when ejaculation does occur, there are techniques, such as Vajroli mudra, to reabsorb semen prior to ejaculation. The much-quoted story that illustrates this technique is that of a seventeenth century Dalai Lama, whose subordinates reproached him for his sexual excesses. Standing on the upper terrace of his palace, he began to urinate. The stream descended from terrace to terrace until it reached the ground. The Dalai Lama then reversed the flow and reabsorbed it into his body. He turned to his subordinates and said, "As you can see, sex for me is quite different than it is for you."

A simpler method of withholding semen during ejaculation is to press the point between the anus and the scrotum, diverting the flow of semen into the bladder. This Daoist technique does not prevent the semen from leaving the testes, but it is said to retain the life force within the body.

"Matsyendrasana increases the appetite by fanning the gastric fire and destroys physical ailments. Kundalini is awakened and the moon made steady."

Hatha Yoga Pradipika

siddhasana
meditate

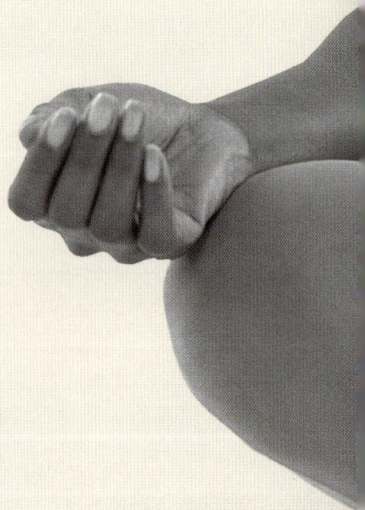

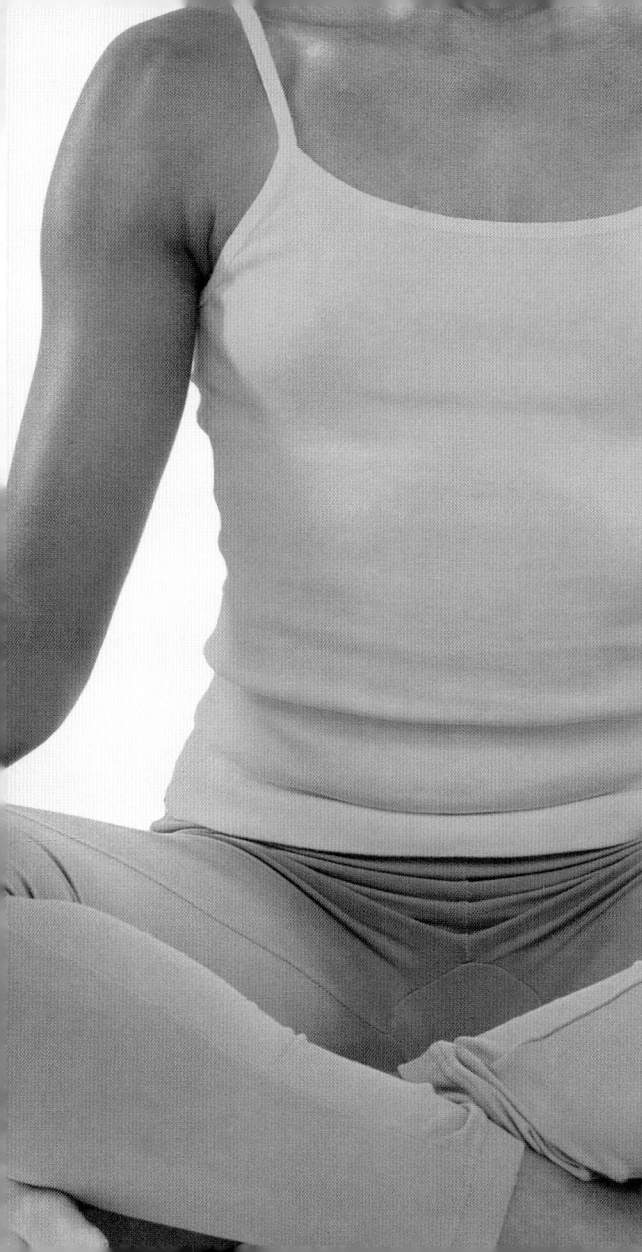

Siddha means perfect,

divine, or accomplished,

and also refers to one

who possesses siddhis,

or supernatural powers.

chapter 8

benefits

Siddhasana does not require the same level of flexibility as the classic Padmasana, commonly known as the lotus posture (see pages 232-3). However, it helps to develop flexibility in the hips, legs, and ankles, and is therefore used as a preparatory exercise for Padmasana. Both postures create the firm seat with the legs locked into place and the straight spine that is needed to maintain long periods of meditation and pranayama practice. However, in this chapter, the poses, be it Siddhasana or Padmasana, are secondary to the mental component of meditation.

MEDITATION AND STRESS

The principle physiological benefit of meditation is its ability to help us control stress. Research conducted by Herbert Benson of the Harvard Medical School's Mind-Body Medical Institute in the late sixties shows that meditation induces a unique physiological state, which Benson dubbed the "relaxation response." Achieving this state allows us to counteract a whole range of mental and physical symptoms caused by stress, including reducing elevated levels of the stress hormones, epinephrin and cortisol, easing anxiety and depression, slowing respiration and heartbeat, and relaxing muscular tension.

meditation guidelines

CLOTHING

Dress appropriately for the season. If you are performing your meditation after posturing or pranayama, both of which have the effect of heating up the body, remember that once immobile, your body will cool down rapidly. On the other hand, an overheated room will encourage drowsiness, so it is better to keep the temperature cool and dress accordingly. Clothing should not constrict your waist or chest.

TIME AND PLACE

Choose the quietest time of your day, which could be early morning before the household gets up, or in mid-morning when everyone has gone out. You may meditate at any time, but avoid times when you are likely to be tired and drowsy, such as mid-afternoon or late evening.

It is possible to meditate anywhere, but as a beginner, you will need a quiet environment, with few colors, sounds, or smells to distract you.

FOOD AND STIMULANTS

It is advisable to allow two hours after a large meal and one hour after a light meal before meditating. Digestion takes a lot of energy and will encourage drowsiness.

In the sixties, many believed that psychoactive drugs, such as LSD and Cannabis, caused an "altered state" similar to meditation. However, in meditation, the mind remains totally alert and conscious, with a high degree of neuronal activity and organization; in contrast, the drugged brain is subject to a gradual loss of consciousness as the brain cells lose their interconnectivity and the mind ultimately reverts to a pre-conscious state.

meditation postures

Meditation techniques have their origins in floor-level cultures of India, China, and Japan. As a result, all meditation postures involve sitting or kneeling on the ground (and occasionally lying, though this encourages fatigue). These postures can prove difficult for many Westerners who do not have the flexibility to hold them for more than a few minutes at a time. As a beginner you may wish to start your practice in a chair, or in modified kneeling or crossed-legged postures. If you are inflexible but would like to sit in Siddhasana, Sukasana, or Ardha Padmasana (see pages 230-231), raise your hips by sitting on a block or a cushion.

The position of the body is also considered vital in meditation because prana, the life force, is said to travel through the nadis and chakras (see page 172). An erect spine will ensure the uninterrupted flow of prana from the base to the crown chakras. In Kundalini yoga, spiritual energy stored at the base of the spine is believed to travel along the central nadi, the Sushumna, which run along the spinal column from the base of the spine to just above the head.

"Place your right foot on your thigh and your left foot on your right thigh with your soles upward, and place the hands on the thighs, with the palms upwards.
This is called Padmasana, the destroyer of all diseases."

Hatha Yoga Pradipika

M

siddhasana—Perfect pose

1 Sit on the floor with your legs outstretched in front of you. Bend your left knee and place your left heel against the perineum and the sole of your foot against the inside of the right thigh.

2 Bend your right knee, and place the outside edge of the right foot where the calf and thigh of the left leg meet, right ankle over left. The heel of your right foot should line up approximately with the navel and be as close to the pubic bone as possible.

3 Rest your hands palms up on the knees, with the thumbs and forefingers touching, or cup your hands in your lap.

4 Maintain a neutral spine. Do not allow you lower back to arch or your upper back to slump. Keep your head erect and balanced on top of your spine.

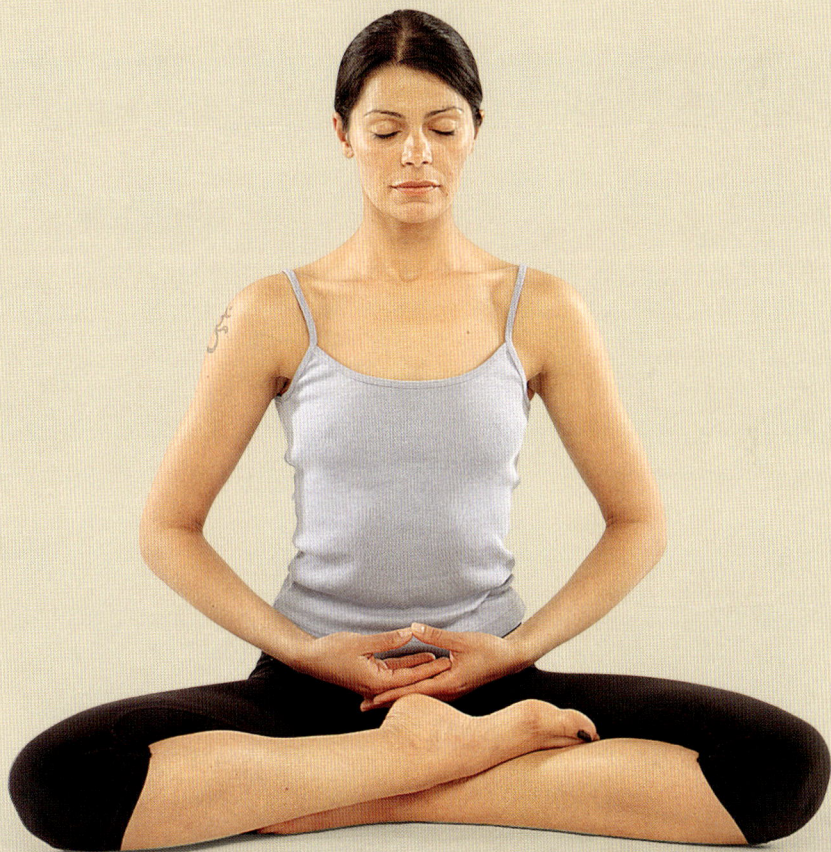

223

E

Sitting

1 If you find it difficult to maintain one of the floor postures with a straight back for any length of time, you may practice meditation sitting on a chair. But it should be a straight-backed chair or stool that will not allow you to slump, and with little or no padding so you do not sink into it.

2 Sit slightly forward so that your back is not in contact with the rear of the chair. Pull the skin of your buttocks to find your sit-bones. Your knees create right angles and your feet are flat on the floor. Keep your arms resting easy, either on your knees or cupped in your lap.

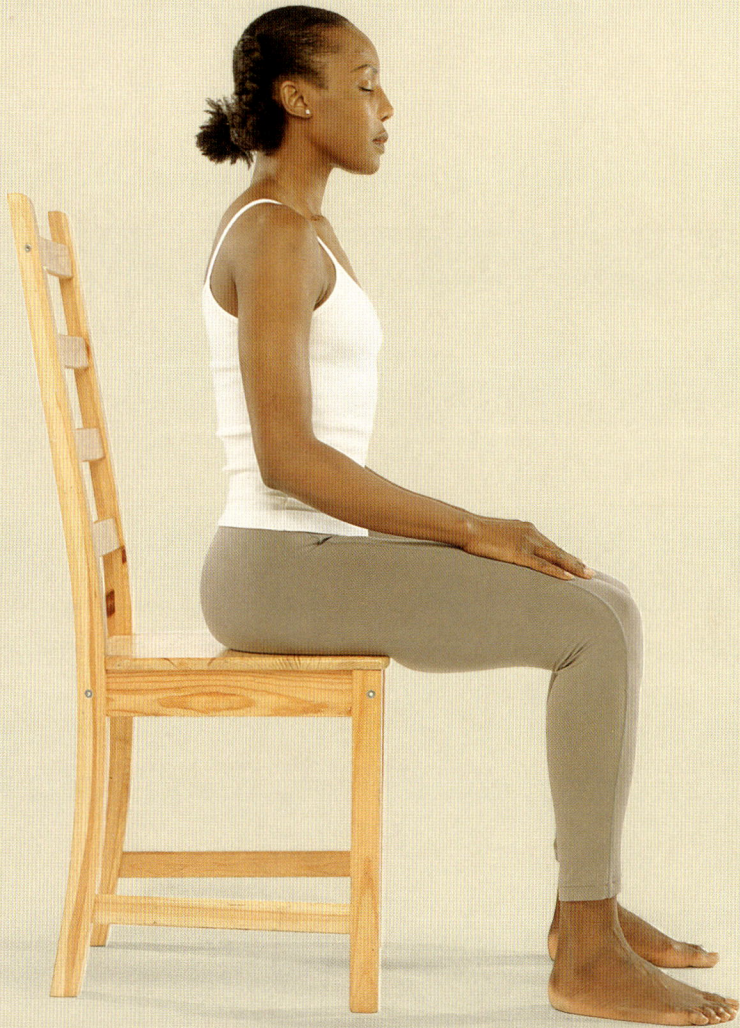

225

E

EASY POSTURE

sukasana—Cross-legged posture

Sit in a comfortable cross-legged posture. Pull the skin of your buttocks to find your sit bones, and let your knees drop. Hold your hands in one of the positions recommended for Siddhasana.

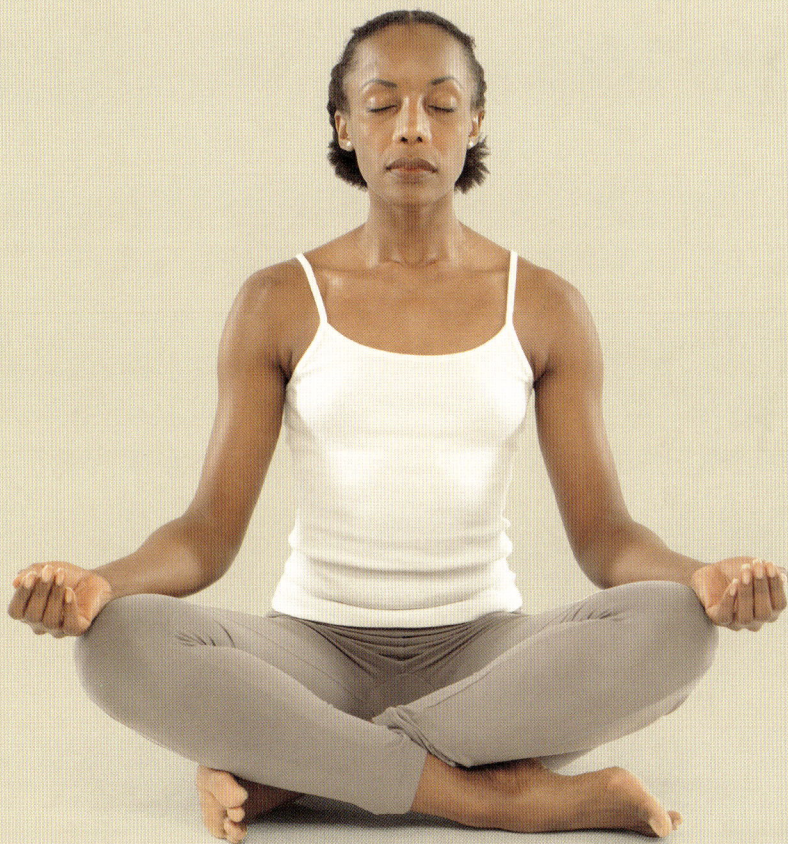

M

MEDIUM POSTURE

vajrasana—Kneeling posture

Known as "seiza" (correct seat) in Japan, this requires good ankle flexibility to be held for any length of time. A good way to practice the pose is to kneel on top of one cushion with a smaller cushion under your buttocks to raise your body and relieve the pressure on your ankles.

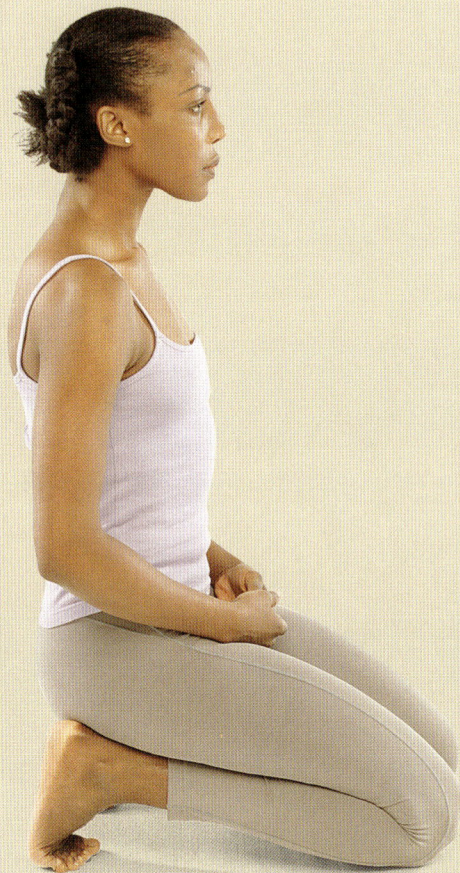

M

ardha-padmasana

Half-lotus posture

In this second preparatory posture for Padmasana, place one of your feet on the top of your opposite thigh, and your other foot is pressed against the perineum. Alternate the feet so that you stretch both sides evenly.

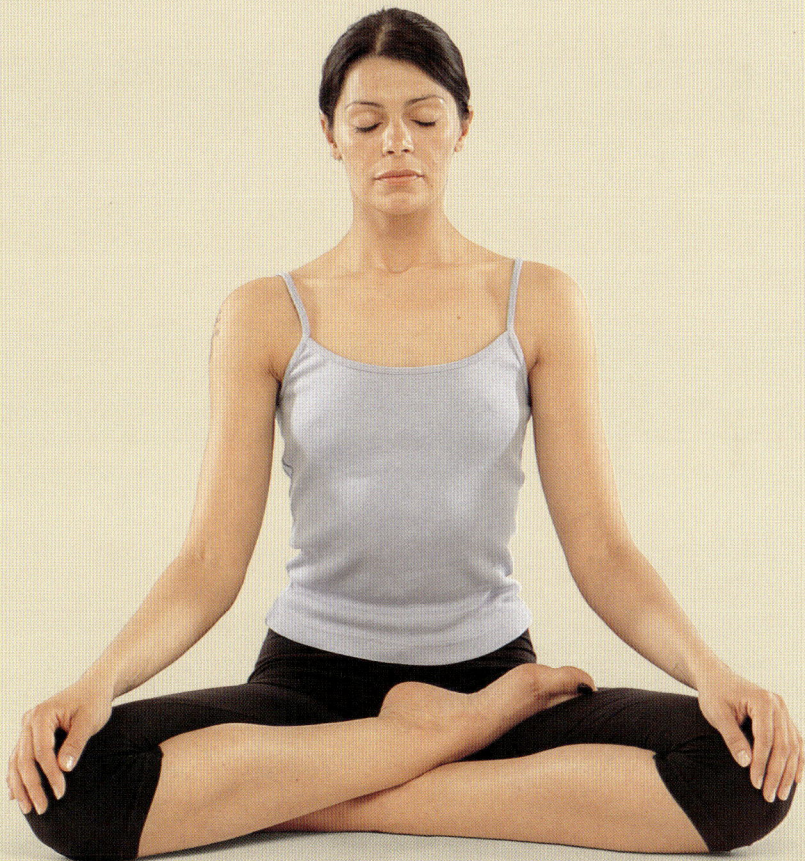

D

padmasana—Lotus posture

1 The classic yoga meditation pose takes its name from the lotus—a symbol of purity because its blooms are unsullied although they grow out of muddy waters.

2 Sit on the floor with your legs stretched straight out in front of you. Bend your right knee and place it on top of your left thigh bringing your left heel as close as possible to your navel.

3 Bend your left knee and place your left foot on top of your right thigh bringing your right heel as close to the navel as possible.

4 Your knees should be on the ground and the soles of your feet should face upward. Hold your hands in one of the positions recommended for Siddhasana.

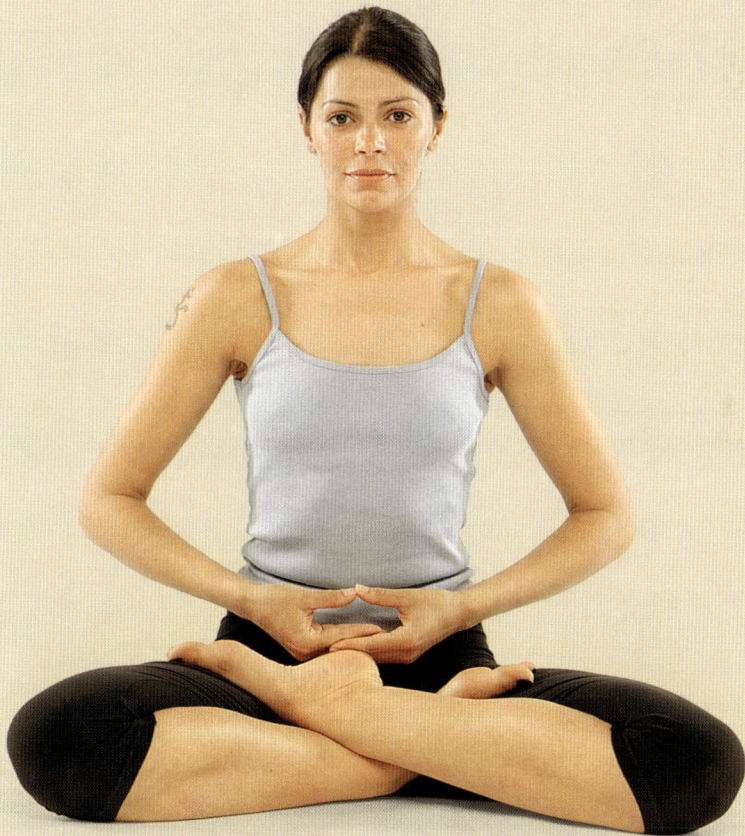

Types of meditation

In a sense, the whole of yoga is a form of meditation that aims to bring the yogi to Samadhi, absorption into Brahman, the eighth and final limb of Patanjali's Ashtanga yoga. Beginning with the postures and pranayama, the body is brought under control. Once this is achieved the mind is controlled by meditation techniques that help the yogi to withdraw the senses from the external world, and turn inward, until he or she can attain the state where the difference between object and subject vanishes.

The meditation techniques given below are alternative ways of achieving the same end. You may find one or more technique preferable for your own practice.

SOUND

Mantra meditation consists of the repetition of a single syllable or phrase to focus the mind. Among the best known is the syllable "Om" (also Aum), which is sometimes translated as "god," but is best understood as representing the impersonal, eternal absolute known as Brahman. Other syllables that can be used are those associated with each chakra. In this case the mantra is associated with visualization as the mind is centered on the chakra within the body.

Another well known mantra, the phrase "Om mani padme Hum" (Om, the jewel in lotus) is repeated just as a Christian might repeat the Lord's Prayer or a Japanese Buddhist the "Namu Amida Butsu" (I entrust myself to the Buddha Amida). My own experience of mantra meditation includes Transcendental Meditation, which was created by the Maharishi Mahesh Yogi (see page 95), in which each student is assigned his or her own mantra. The advantage of sound-based meditation for a beginner is that by engaging one of the major senses it is much easier to calm the mind.

Another more difficult form of meditation using sound is Nada, listening to internal and mystic sounds, such as one's own breathing and heartbeat, and in some traditions, listening to the mystic sounds made by the Universe itself, which are akin to the Mediaeval Christian "music of the spheres."

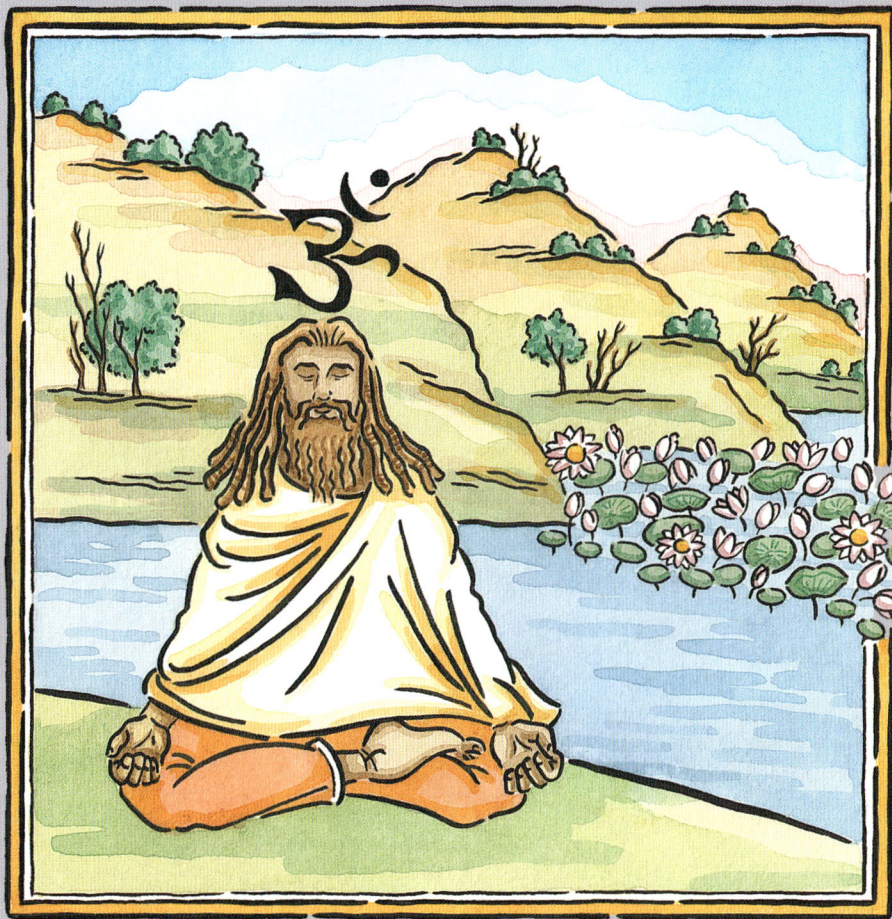

SIGHT

As the pre-eminent human sense, sight is used in various yoga techniques, such as the Trataka cleansing technique (see page 120). In classic Yantra and Mandala meditation, sacred symbols (yantras) and diagrams (mandalas) are used as the focus of the mind. The diagrams may vary from extremely simple geometrical shapes, such as a circle or triangle, to extremely intricate, colorful designs that include representations of the Hindu deities.

The images of the Hindu gods (or of the religion that you follow) or of inspirational spiritual figures, such as Mahatma Gandhi or Mother Theresa, can be used as the focus of meditation. Allow their boundless wisdom and compassion to fill your mind as you concentrate on their physical image. A related technique is visualization in which an object, image, or person is constructed in your mind's eye. A visualization technique also employed in Daoism is to imagine the flow of prana into the body, and to direct it through the nadis to the chakras.

"The yogi in highest meditation is a void within and void without. Like a pitcher in the ocean, full within and without."

Hatha Yoga Pradipika

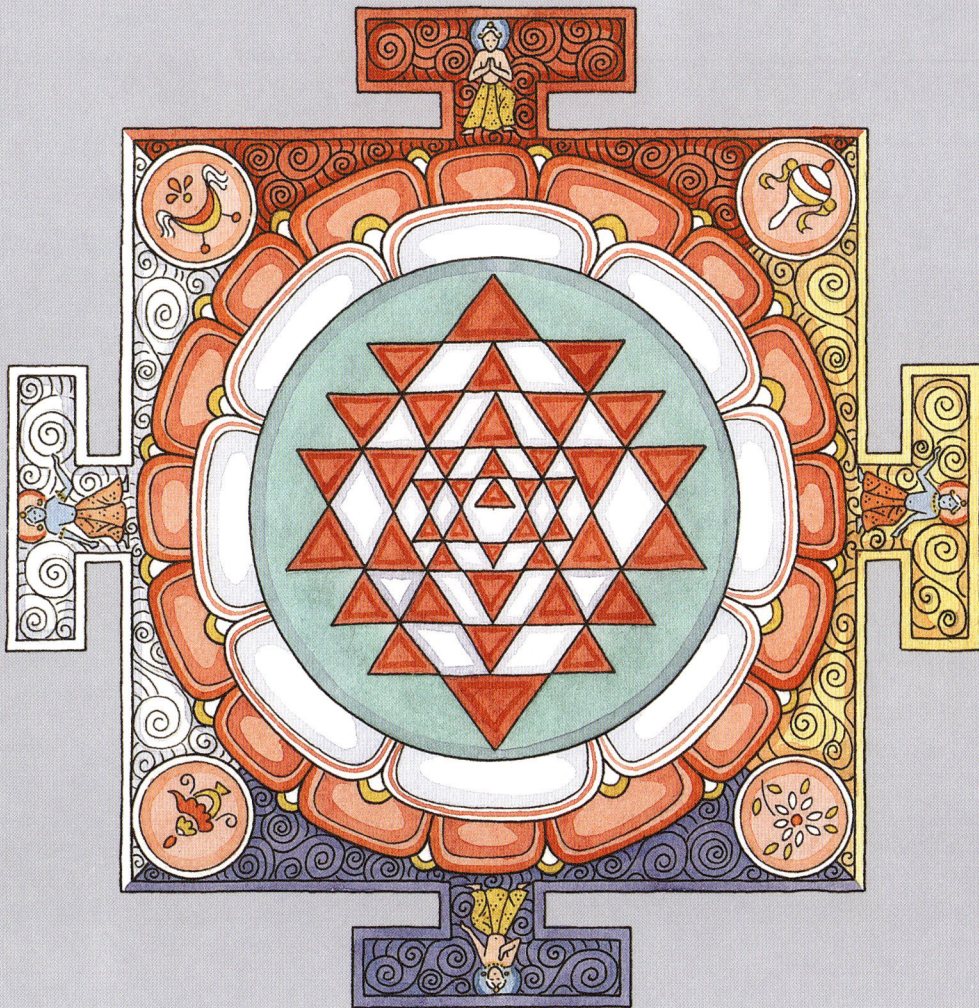

Concentration

Practicing meditation when the focus is on the self is considered to be the most difficult. One such technique is zazen, Zen Buddhist sitting, which originated in Dhyana, meditation, the seventh limb of Patanjali's Ashtanga yoga. Zazen is deceptively simple in its practice: students are instructed to sit or kneel on cushions facing the wall, eyes open, with their minds empty. During a two hour session, they will sit for between twenty and forty minutes, with 10–minute breaks for walking meditation. Zazen is difficult precisely because there is no external stimulus to hold the mind. At the beginner stage, students are encouraged to count their breaths in cycles of ten, starting again if they lose count or their attention wanders.

> "The real meaning of yoga is deliverance from pain and sorrow."
>
> *Hatha Yoga Pradipika*

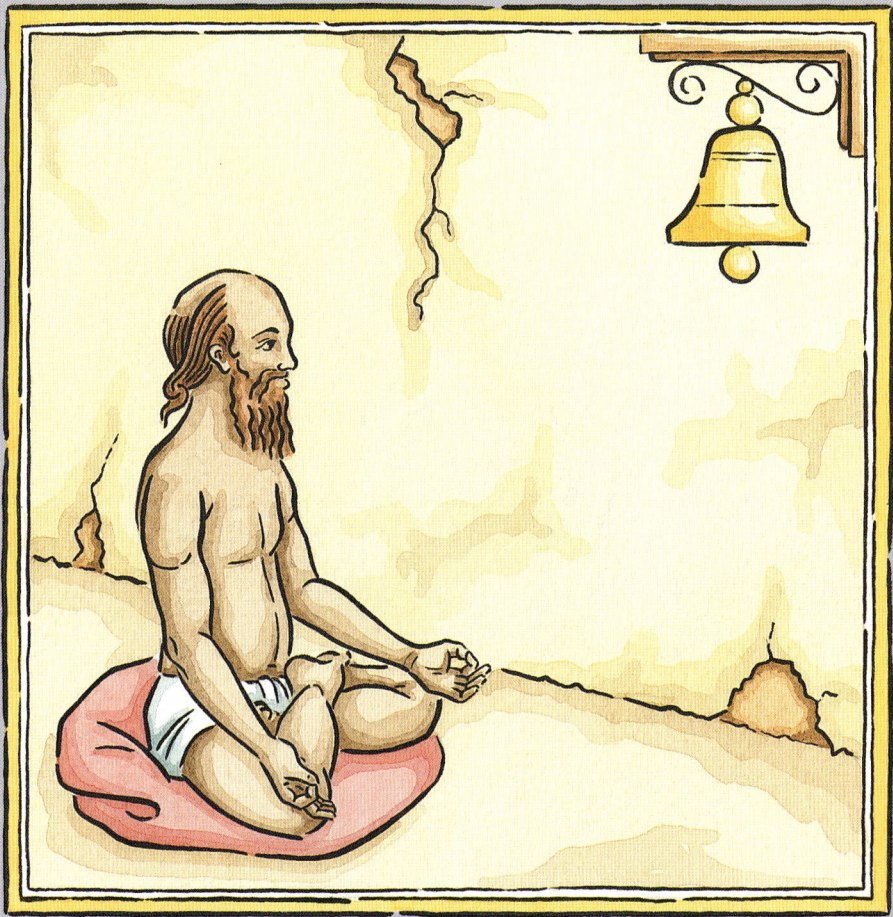

Hinduism

Hinduism, like Christianity, is monotheistic, believing in a single transcendent godhead, Brahman. To understand the relationship between this monotheistic philosophy and the large pantheon of Hindu gods and goddesses, imagine that instead of replacing Greek and Roman paganism, Christianity had just been grafted onto it, so that the once all powerful gods and goddesses of Olympus, had become different aspects of the one god revealed by Jesus Christ.

One of the beliefs shared by all Hindus is that the sum of one's actions in life (one's karma) determines whether we will be reincarnated at a higher or lower level of life. The aim of Hinduism is Moksha, liberation from rebirth, and Samadhi, absorption into the final unchanging reality of Brahman. As we have seen, this release may be achieved within Hinduism through one of many paths, including good works (Karma yoga), devotion to a particular god (Bhakti yoga), meditation (Raja yoga), and, of course, posturing (Hatha yoga).

HINDU GODS

The Hindu trinity, the Trimurti, of Brahma, Vishnu, and Shiva, represents the creative, sustaining, and destructive forces of the universe. Brahma, who is not to be confused with Brahman, the abstract conception of godhead found in the Upanishads (see page 242), emerges from the cosmic egg to begin the cyclical process of creation and destruction of the world. His four heads and arms represent the four Vedas, castes, and yugas (ages of the world). Vishnu is known as the Preserver. His ten manifestations, or avatars, include Rama and Krishna. Shiva is known as the Destroyer, but he also represents the principle of generation symbolized by the lingam (phallus). In addition to the Trimurti, Hindus also worship a number of goddesses who are seen to be different aspects of a single Great Goddess. The popularity of the various gods has waxed and waned with the centuries. Brahma, the Hindu Zeus, was replaced in popularity by Shiva and Vishnu in the seventh century.

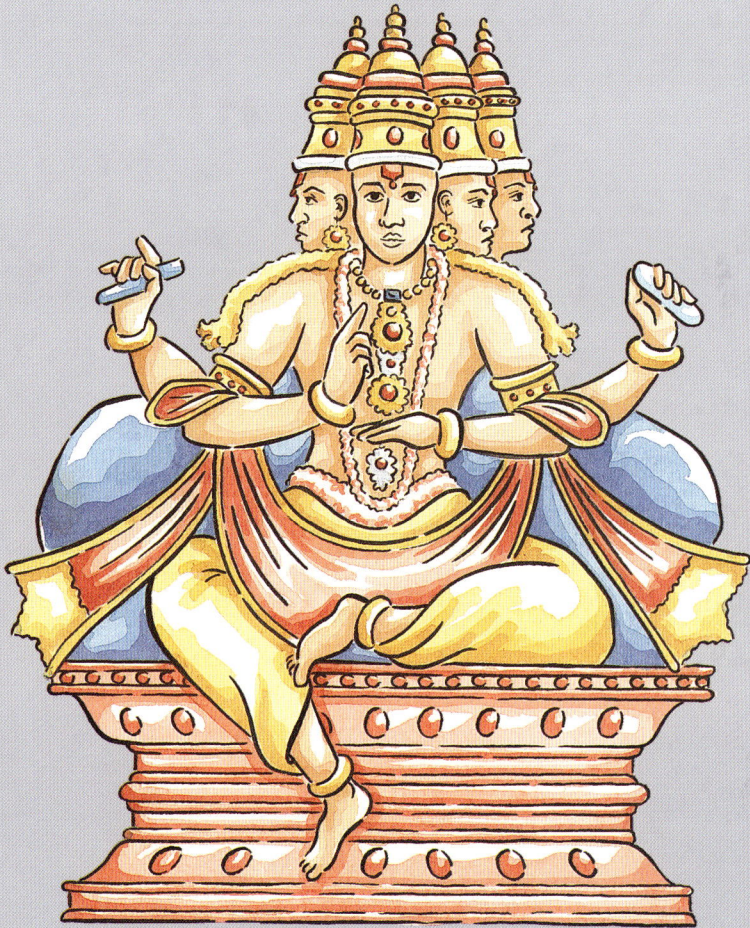

Hindu classics

VEDAS AND UPANISHADS

Believed to be eternal and of divine origin, the Vedas form the scriptural basis for Hinduism. They are the oldest texts of Hinduism, composed between the eighteenth and fourth century B.C.E. The four collections of the Vedas are the Rig Veda, Sama Veda, Yajur Veda, and Atharva Veda. They are divided into the Mantras (verses of invocation and praise), and Brahmanas (rituals and commentaries on the background of the Mantras).

The Upanishads were later added to these. The word upanishad means "esoteric teaching." They consist of about two hundred metaphysical writings, produced as commentaries on the Vedas, and date from between the eighth and fourth century B.C.E. The spirit of the Upanishads is best expressed by its description of Brahman, the ultimate reality. When asked to define Brahman, the sage replies, "Neti, neti (Not this, not this)!" and later explains, "Tat tvam asi (Thou art that)."

Bhagavad Gita

Considered to be an Upanishad, the Bhagavad Gita (The Song of the Bhagava; second century BCE) is part of a larger collection of stories, the Mahabharata, which is the epic tale of the conflict between the warrior Arjuna and members of his own clan. His conscience troubled by the idea of making war on his own kin, Arjuna turns for advice to his charioteer, Krishna, who is the eighth incarnation of Vishnu. At first Krishna's advice is pragmatic, but this is only a preamble to a more spiritual path, and the text becomes an exposition of Karma yoga (yoga of action), Jnana yoga (yoga of wisdom), and Bhakti yoga (yoga of devotion).

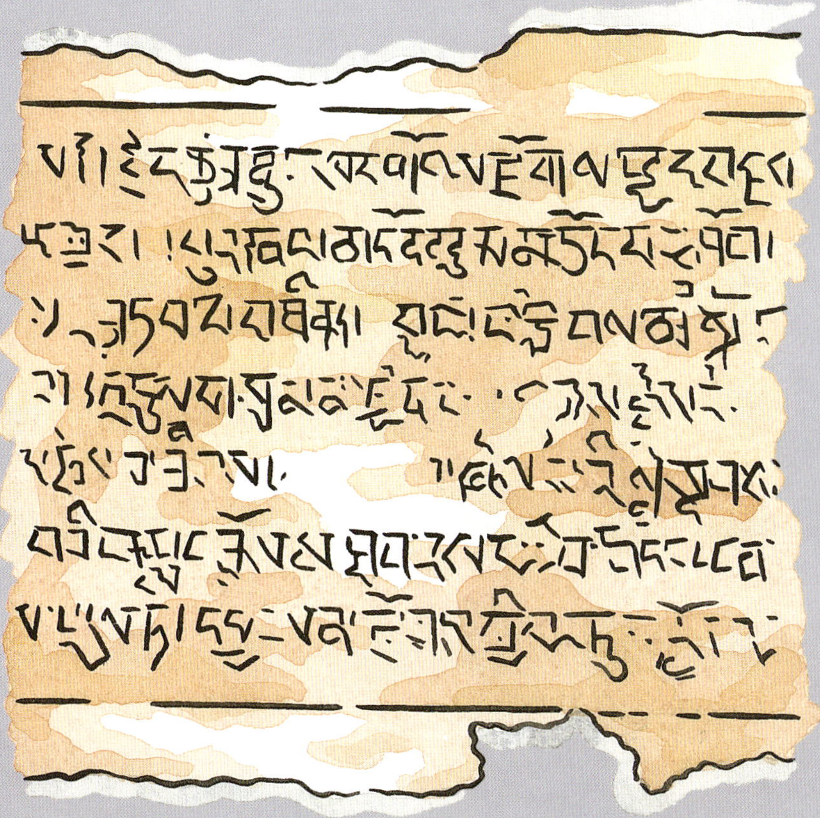

exercise
programs

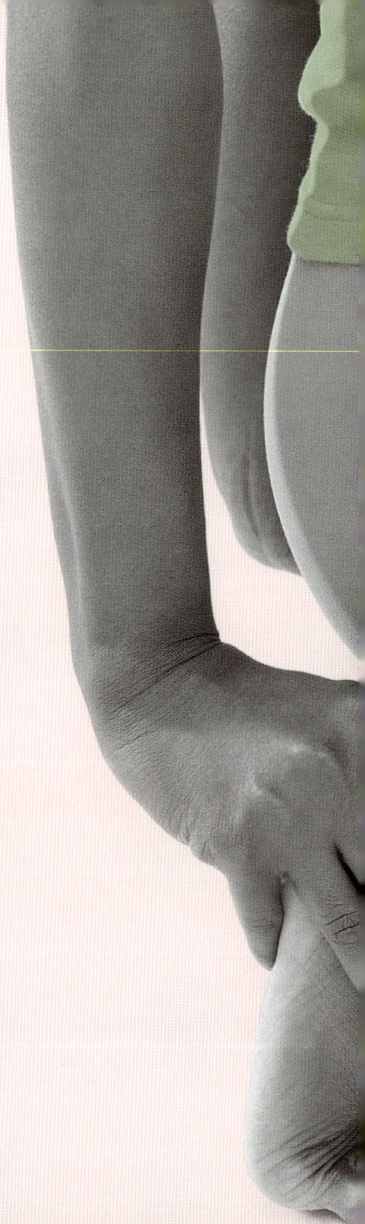

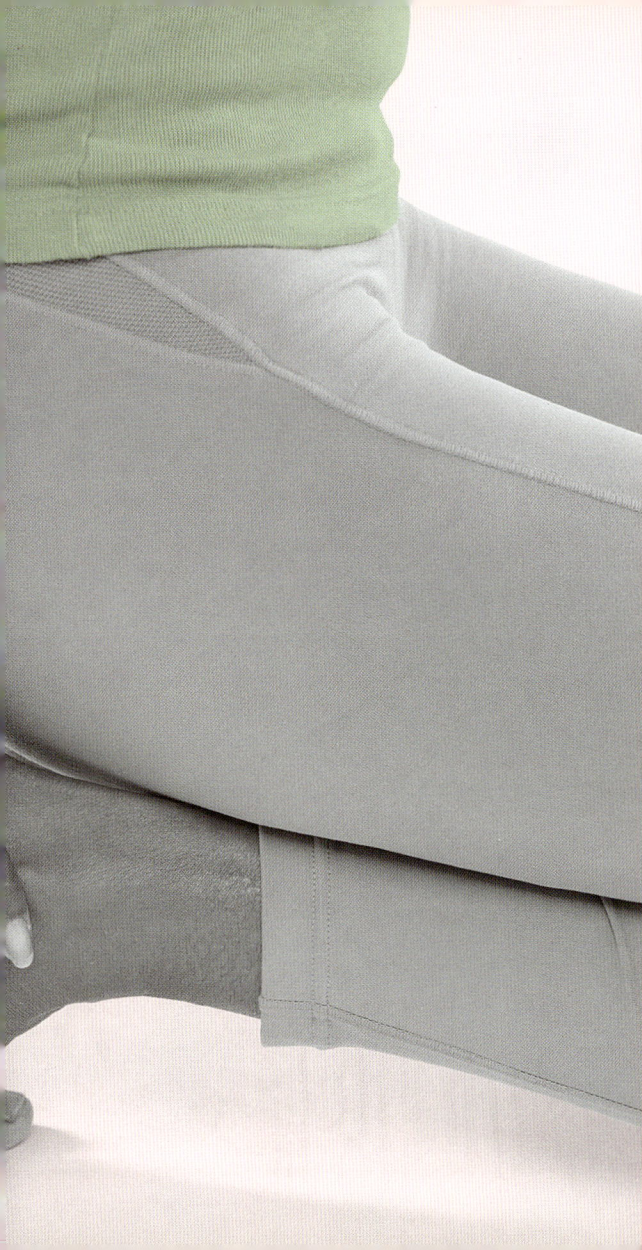

chapter 9

warm up

Hold each posture for three to five breaths unless otherwise instructed. Stretch slowly and smoothly without any jerky movements.

Perform the following sequence:

1 Head roll
2 Arm stretch
3 Cat posture
4 Wrist stretch
5 Seated twist
6 Squat and straighten
7 Ankle and toe stretch
8 Spinal rock

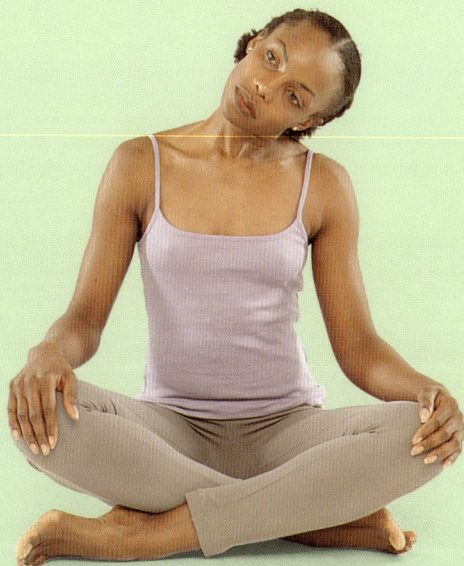

Head roll

Turn your head to the side and roll it down to the front, and back to the side again. It is not advisable to tilt and roll your head back. Complete ten times switching direction after five.

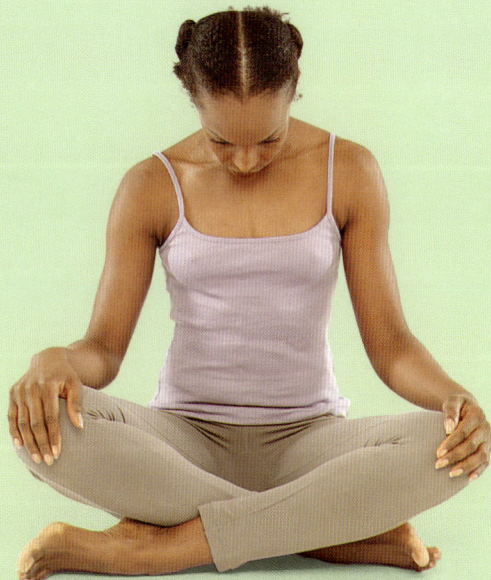

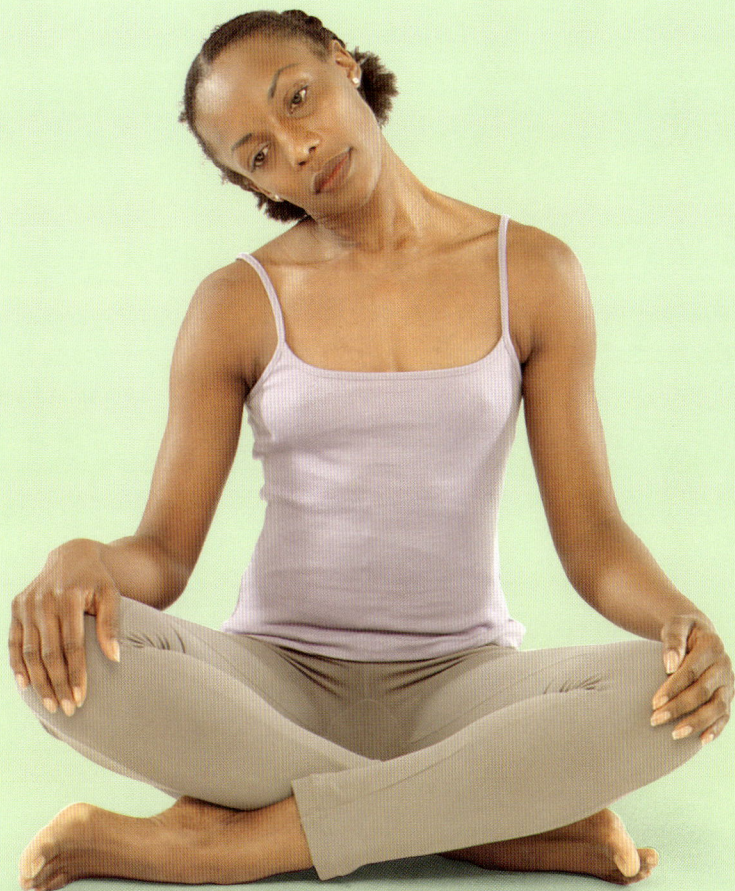

Arm stretch

Put your left hand over your shoulder and your right hand behind your back and try to catch hold of them. Hold for 3-5 breaths. Switch hands and repeat.

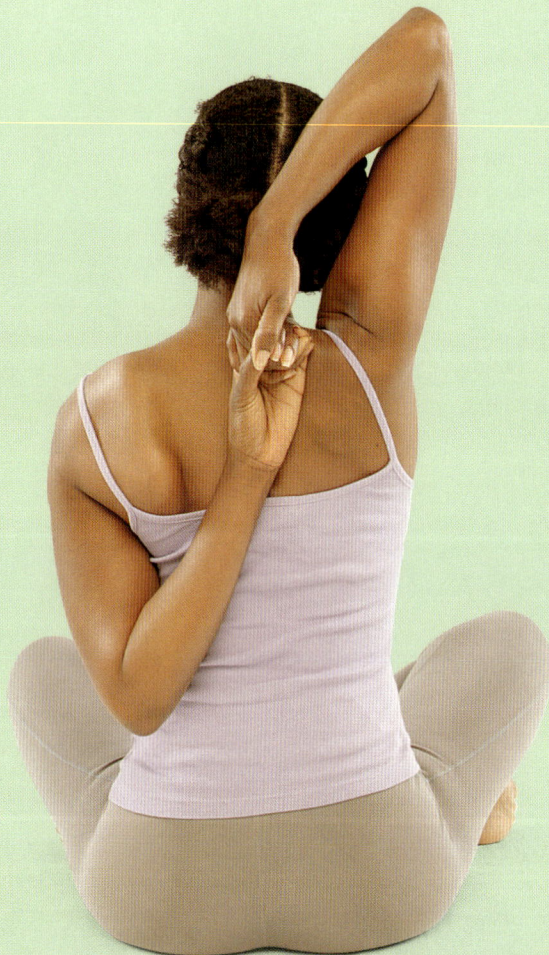

Cat posture

Kneeling on all fours with your hands under your shoulders, hollow your spine and tilt your head back. Then, round your spine, and drop your head. Hold each stage for 3-5 breaths.

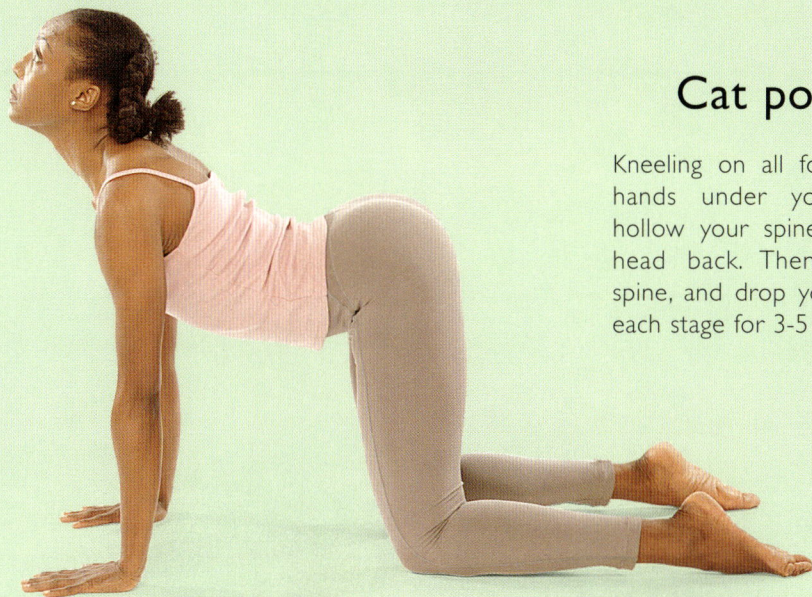

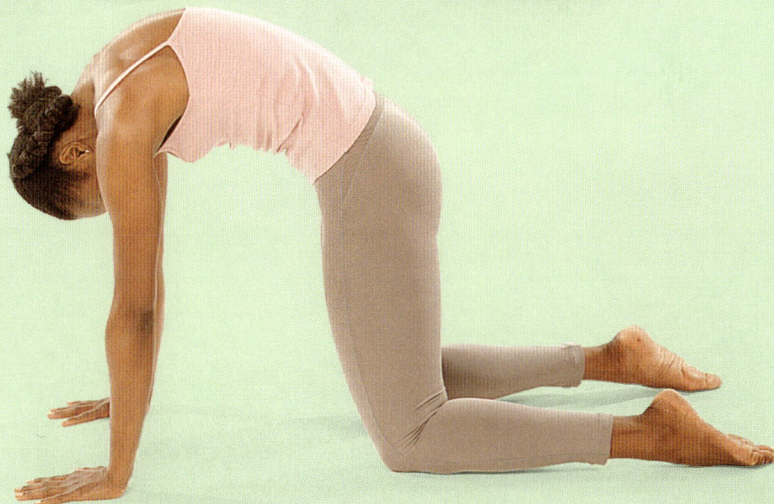

251

Wrist stretch

Kneel with your hands, palms down, in front of you, fingers pointing toward you. If you find it comfortable, put all your weight on your hands and pull back, keeping your palms flat on the floor.

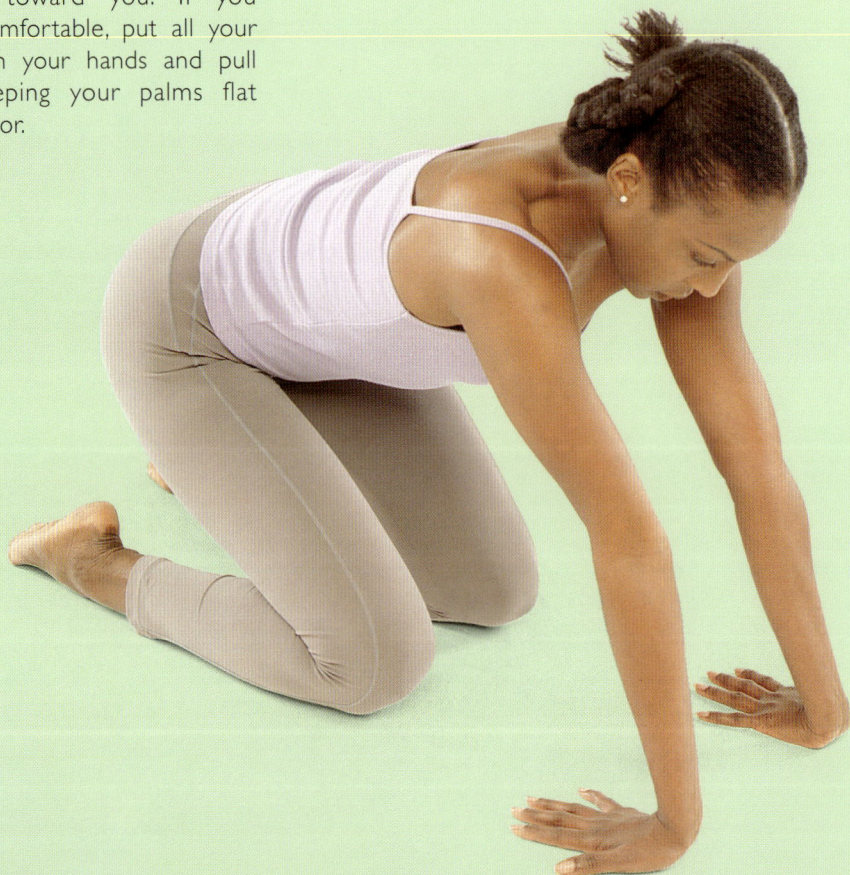

Seated twist

Sitting cross-legged or in a chair, put your right hand on your left knee, and twist the body to the left. Look over your shoulder. Hold for 3-5 breaths, and repeat on the other side.

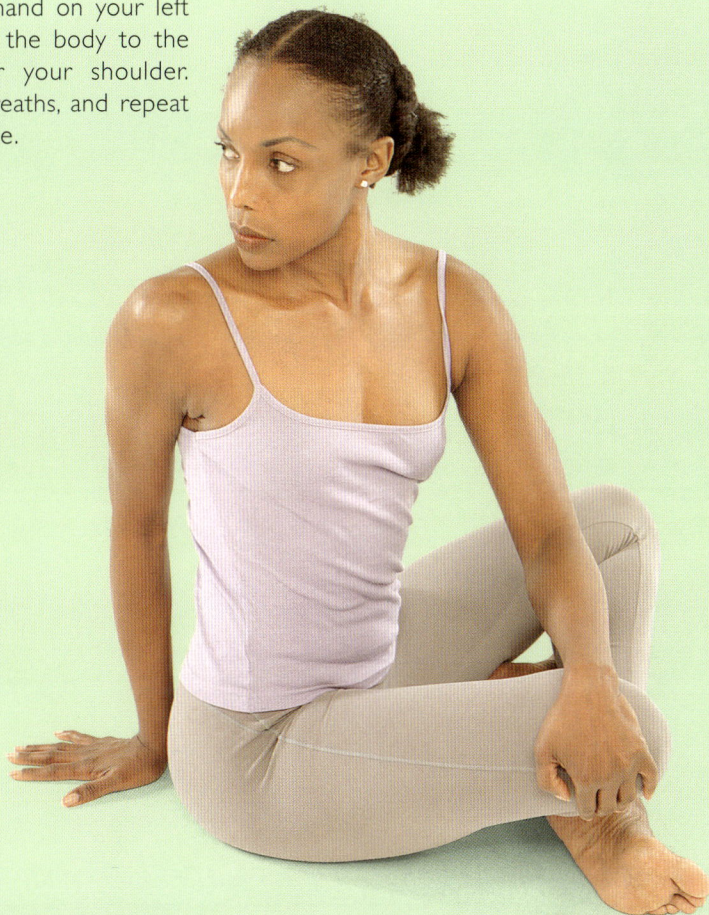

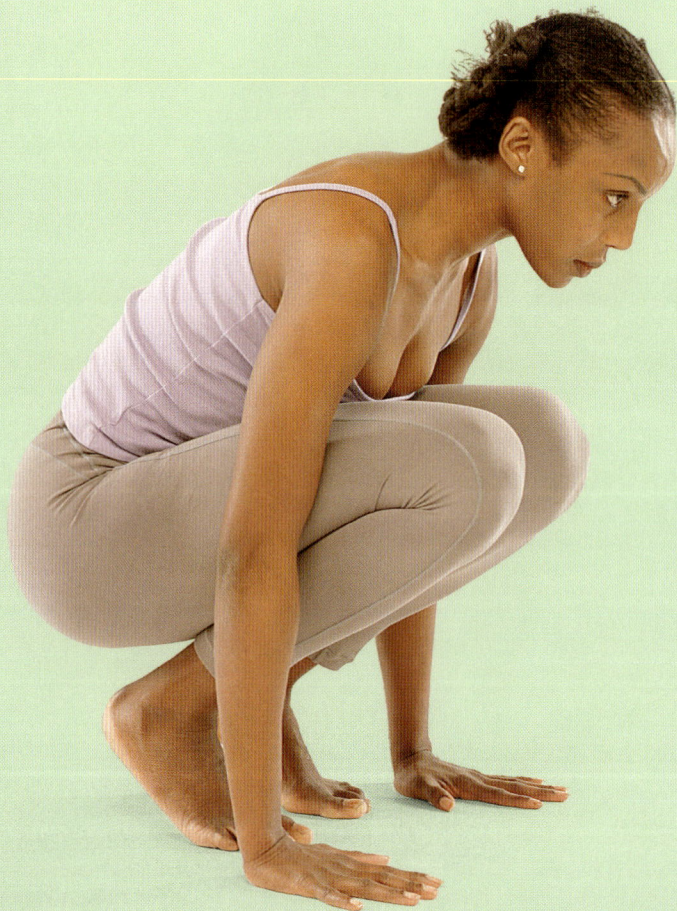

Squat and straighten

Squat down, placing your hands on the floor in front of you. Keeping your knees slightly bent and your palms or fingertips on the floor, straighten your legs. Repeat five times.

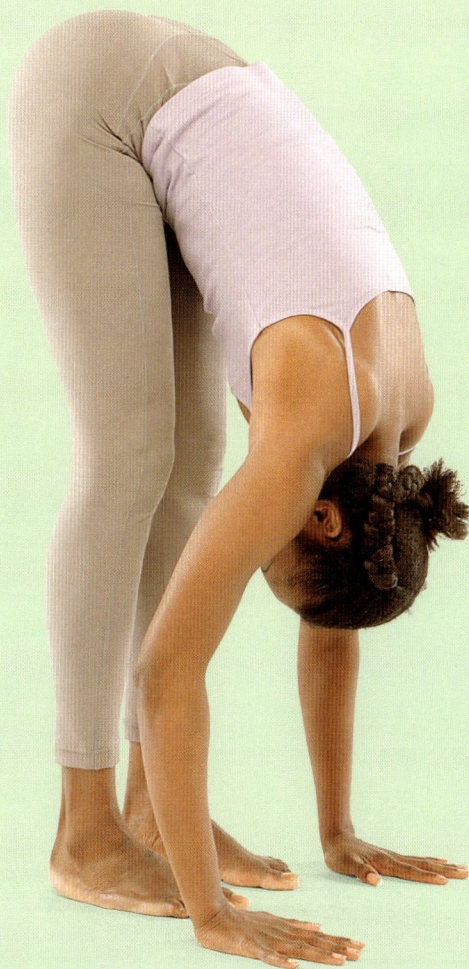

Ankle and
toe stretch

Kneel so that your weight is
resting on your toes.

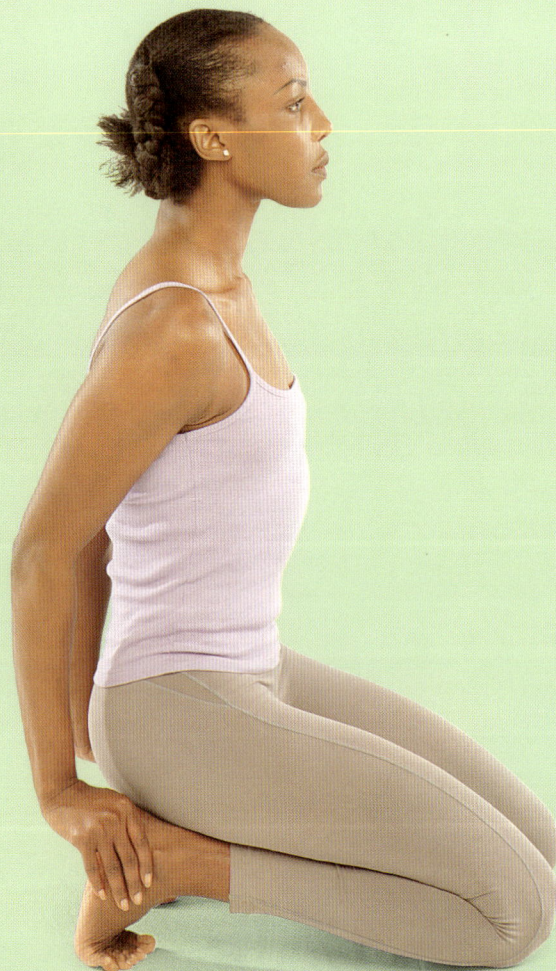

Spinal rock

Lying on your back on the floor, hug your knees to your chest and begin to rock your body so that you roll up and over. Start slow and rock yourself up to a sitting position after 10 repetitions.

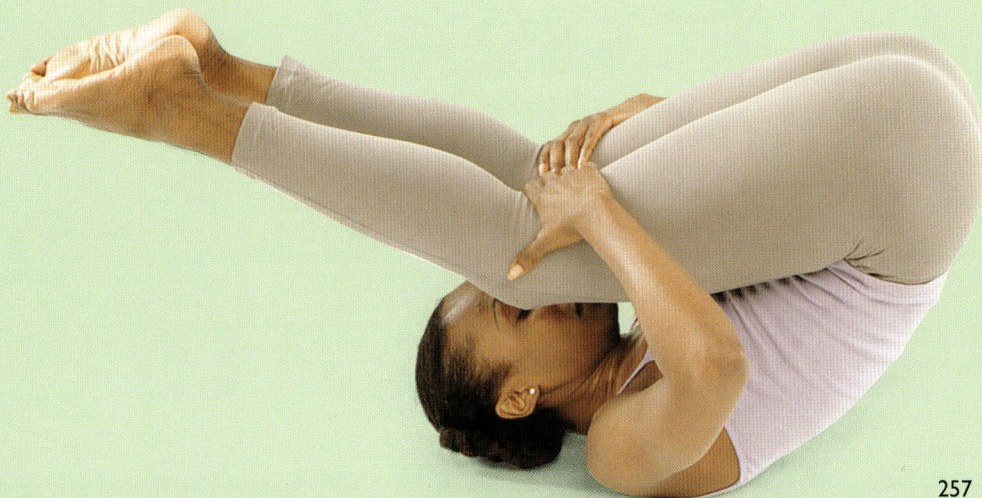

short program

Hold each posture for three to five breaths unless otherwise instructed. Stretch slowly and smoothly without any jerky movements.

Perform the following sequence:

1 Corpse posture
2 Mountain posture
3 Tree posture
4 Serpent posture
5 Shoulder stand
6 Half spinal twist
7 Perfect posture

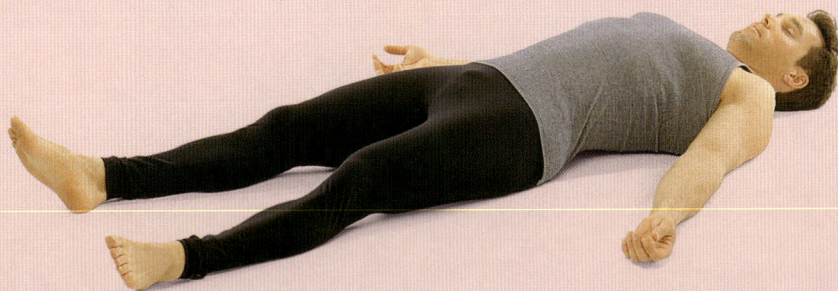

Corpse posture

Perform the progressive relaxation. For full instructions see page 276.

Mountain posture

Stand for 10 full abdominal breaths. Try to identify and relax any remaining areas of tension in your body. For full instructions see pages 82–3.

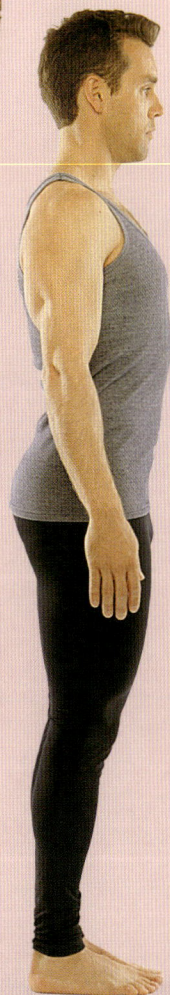

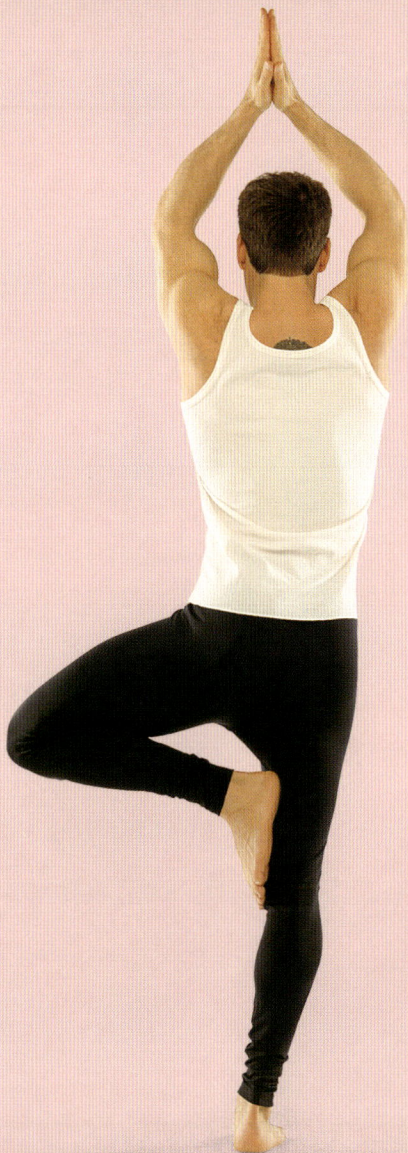

Tree posture

Hold for 3-5 breaths. For full instructions see pages 110–11.

Serpent posture

Hold for 3-5 breaths. For full instructions see pages 132–3.

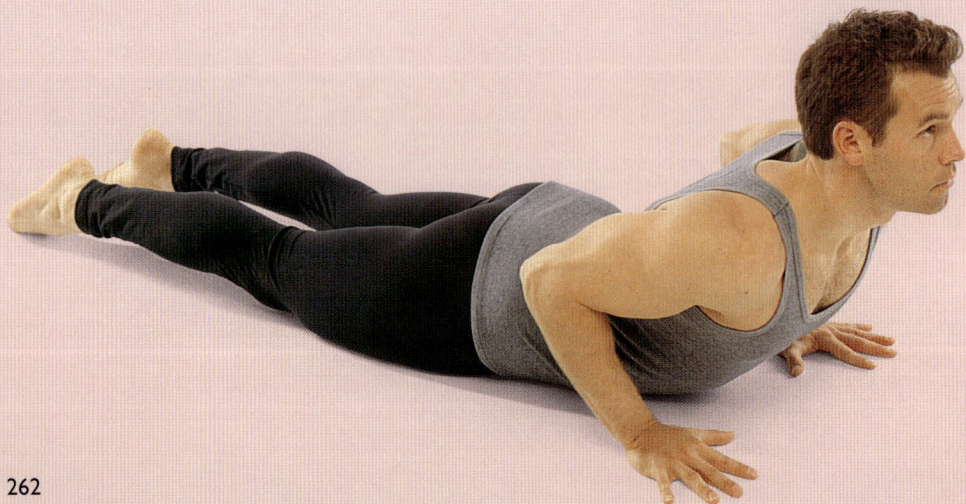

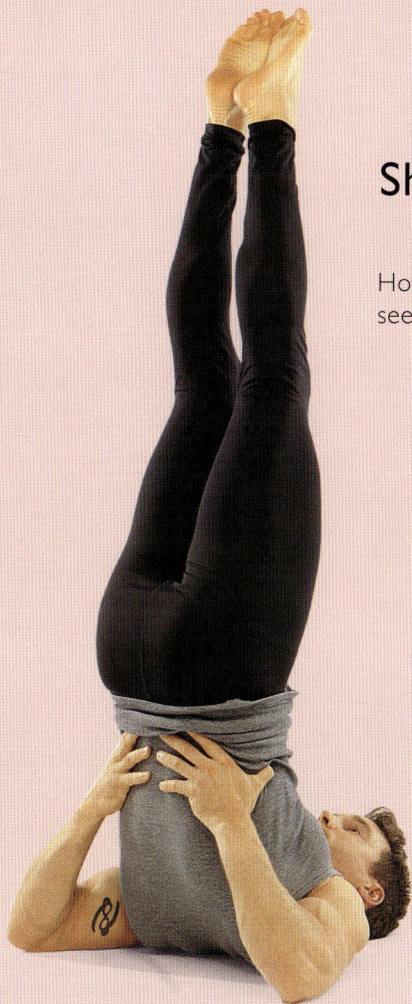

Shoulder stand posture

Hold for 3-5 breaths. For full instructions see pages 158–61.

Half spinal twist posture

Hold for 3-5 breaths. For full instructions see pages 194–5.

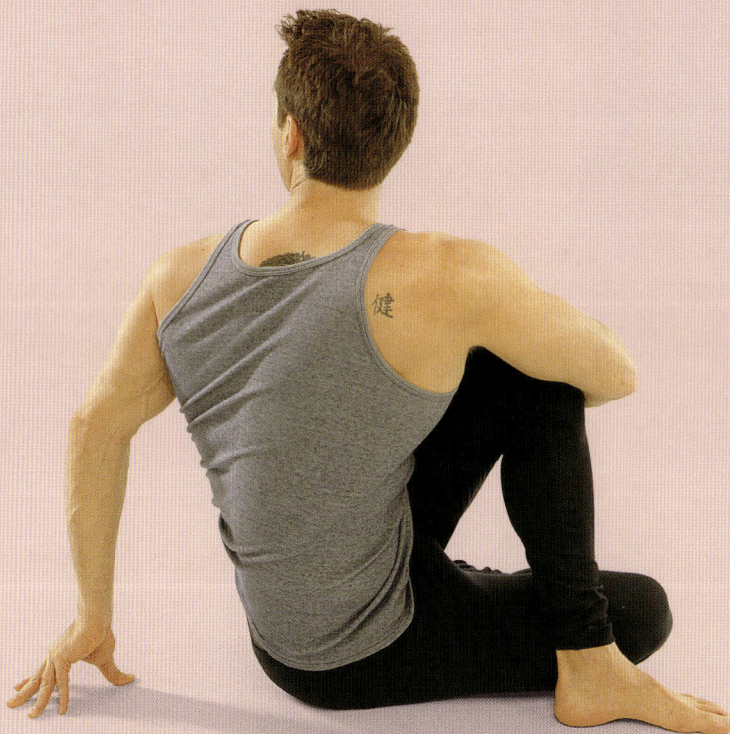

Perfect posture

Sit for at least five minutes using one of the meditation techniques from Chapter Eight. Switch legs if the posture becomes uncomfortable. For full instructions see pages 222–23.

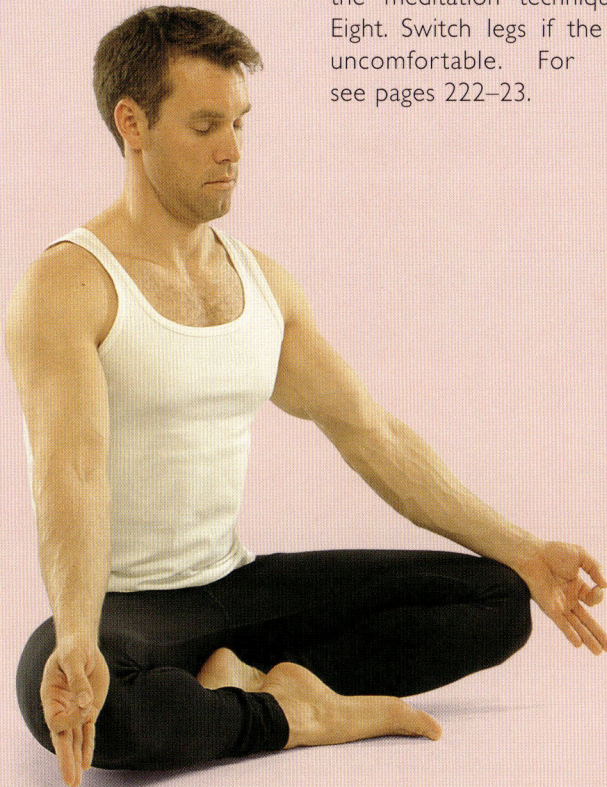

pranayama
program

After performing the progressive relaxation, find a comfortable sitting position. Relax the shoulders and arms. Rest your hands on your thighs, palms up. Keep your back straight, neck long, and your head upright, chin in. Relax your face, and close your eyes.

Perform the following sequence:

1. Corpse posture
2. Cleansing breath
3. Abdominal breathing
4. Victorious breath
5. Alternate nostril breathing

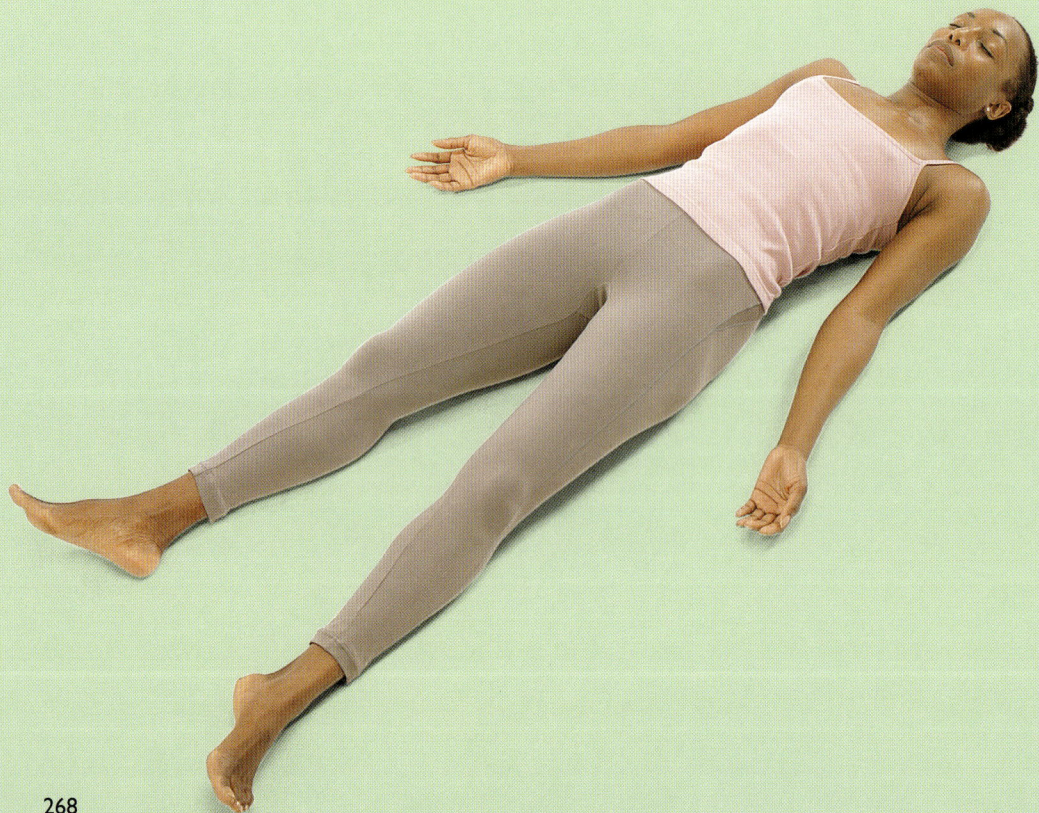

Corpse posture

Perform the progressive relaxation. For full instructions see page 276.

Cleansing breath

Perform two sets of 20 rapid breaths. After each set, perform two breath cycles of Abdominal breathing. See page 66 for full instruction.

Victorious breath

Ten full breath cycles with a 3-5 second kumbhaka (retention between in and out-breath). See page 67 for full instruction.

Abdominal breathing

Ten full breath cycles with a 3-5 second kumbhaka (retention between in and out-breath). For full instructions see page 65.

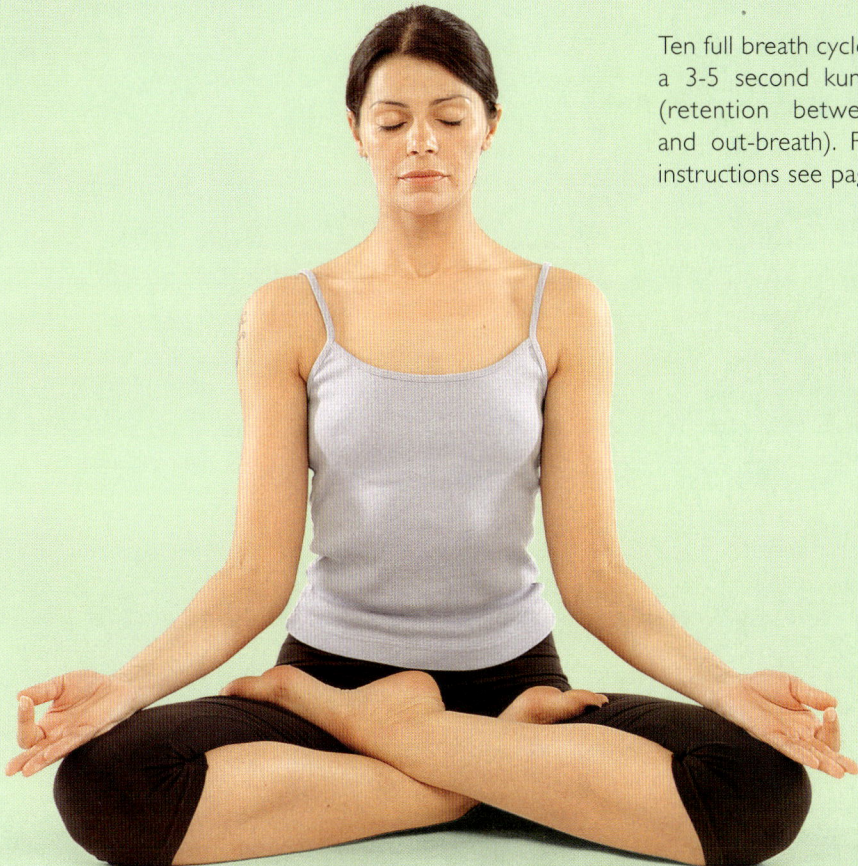

Alternative nostril breathing

Perform 10 full breath cycles. For full instructions see pages 68–9.

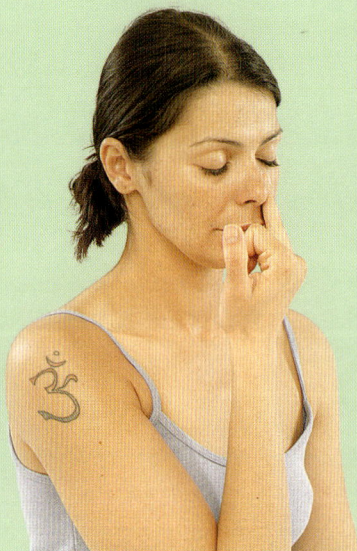

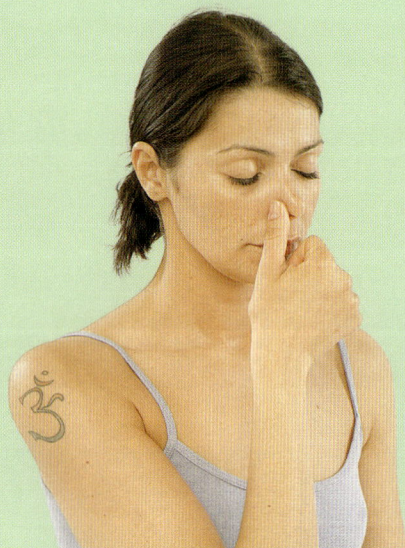

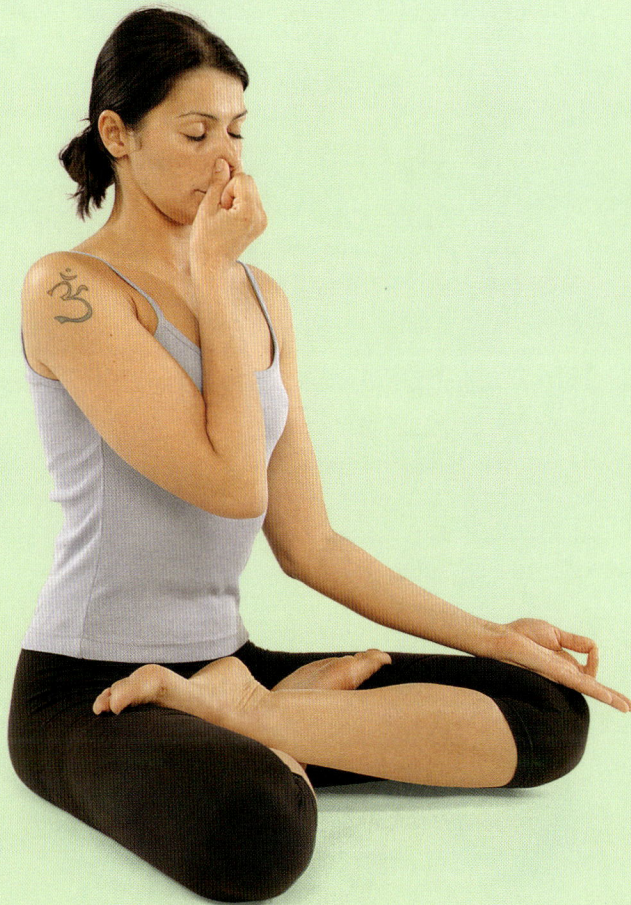

standard program

Hold each posture for three to five breaths unless otherwise instructed. Stretch slowly and smoothly without any jerky movements.

Perform the following sequence:

1 Corpse posture
2 Warrior posture I
3 Warrior posture II
4 Triangle posture
5 Tree posture
6 One leg balance posture
7 Serpent posture
8 Shoulder stand posture
9 Plough posture
10 Fish posture
11 Wheel posture
12 Headstand posture
13 Child posture
14 Supine twist posture
15 Half spinal twist posture
16 Half-lotus or Lotus posture

Corpse posture

Perform the progressive relaxation and 10 cycles of Supine Abdominal breathing. For full instructions on these techniques, see pages 32–6, and page 65.

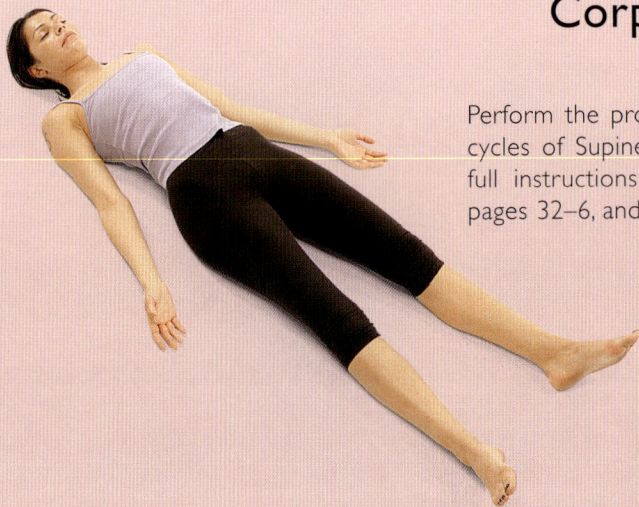

Warrior I posture

For full instructions see pages 84–5.

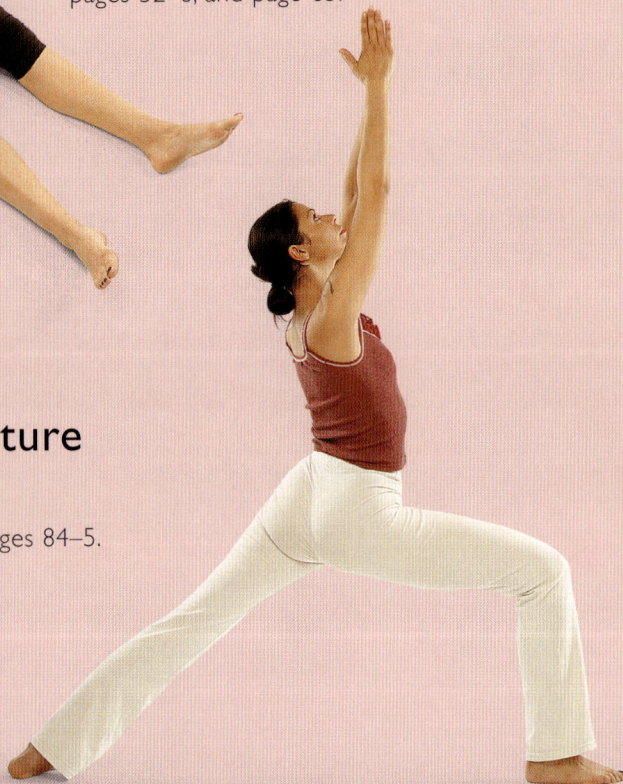

Warrior II posture

For full instructions see page 86–7.

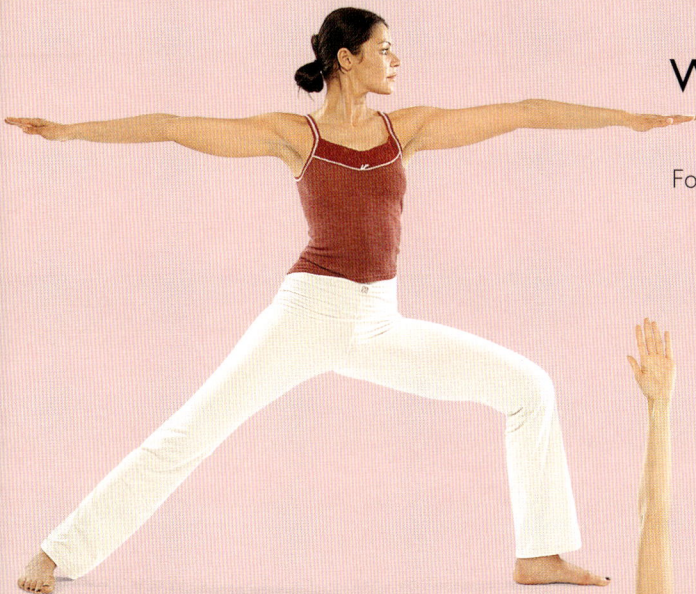

Triangle posture

For full instructions see pages 90–1.

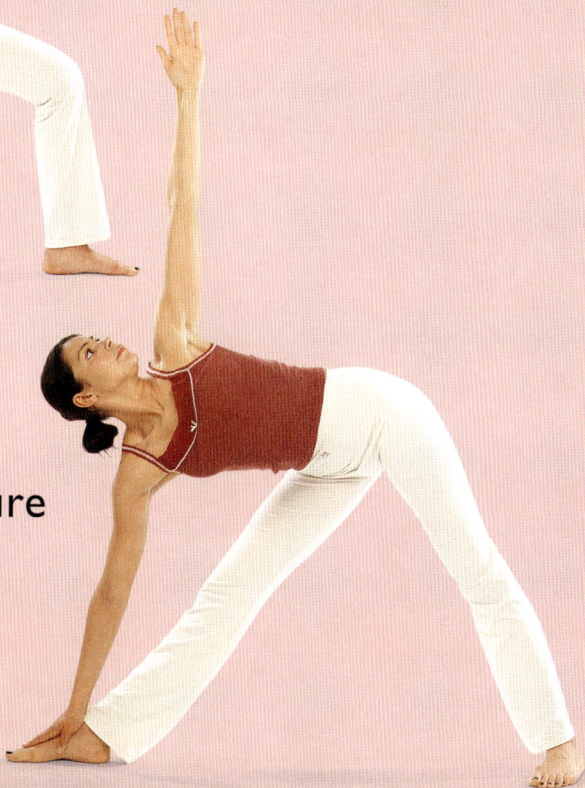

Tree posture

For full instructions see
pages 110–11.

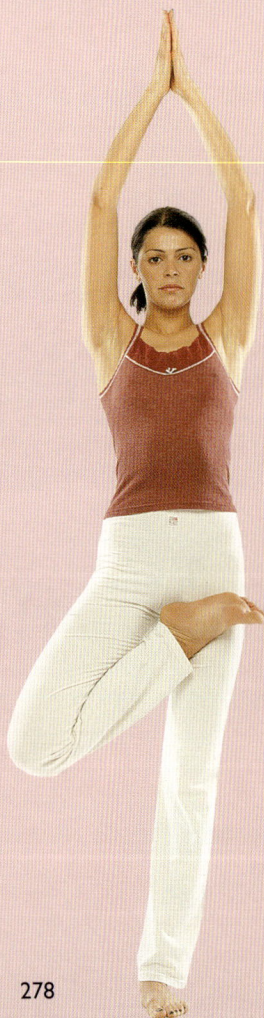

One leg balance

posture

For full instructions
see pages 114–15.

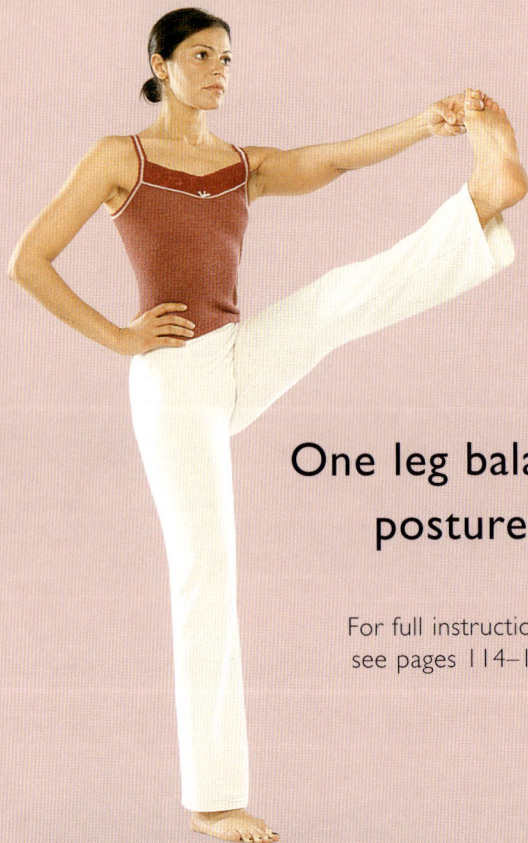

Serpent posture

For full instructions see pages
132–3.

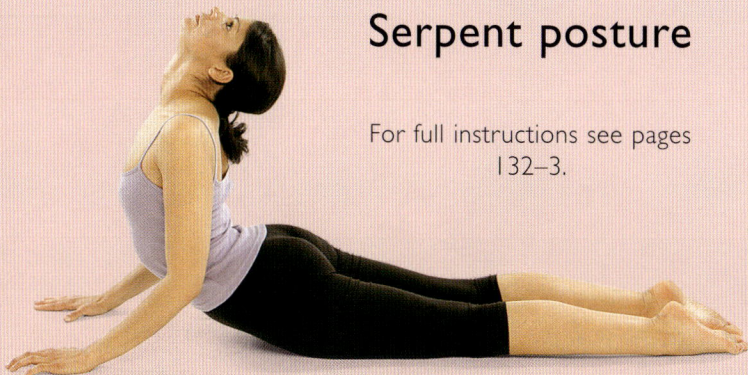

Shoulder stand

posture

For full instructions
see pages 158–61.

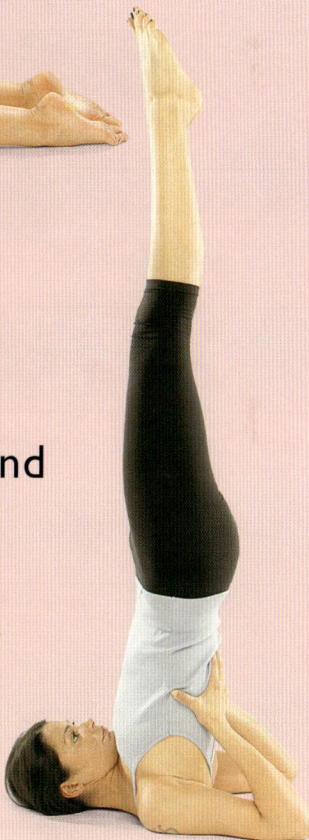

Plough posture

For full instructions
see pages 162–3.

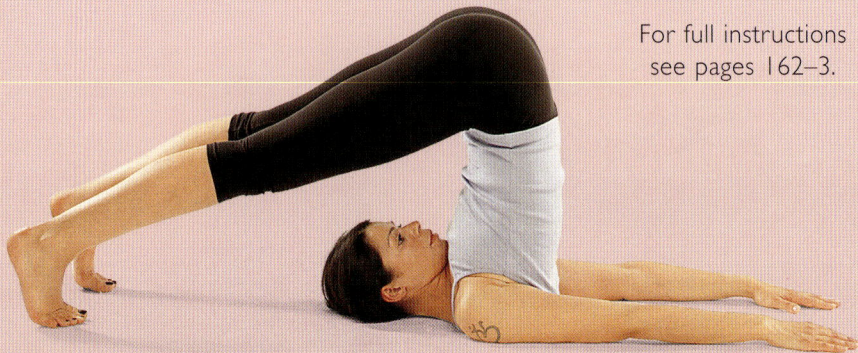

Fish posture

For full instructions
see pages 136–7.

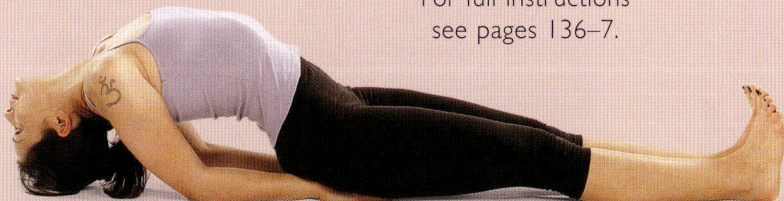

Wheel posture

For full instructions
see pages 144–5.

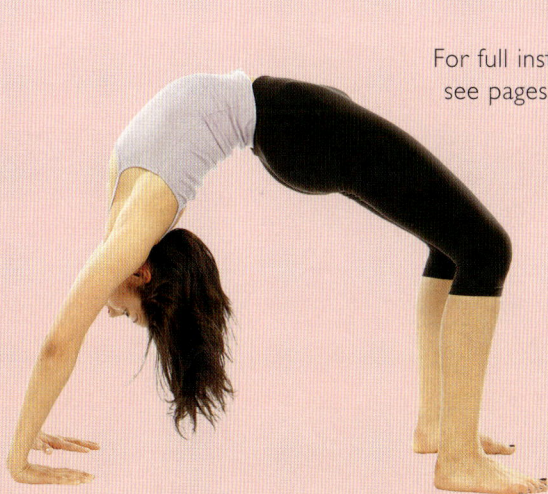

Headstand posture

For full instructions
see pages 164–7.

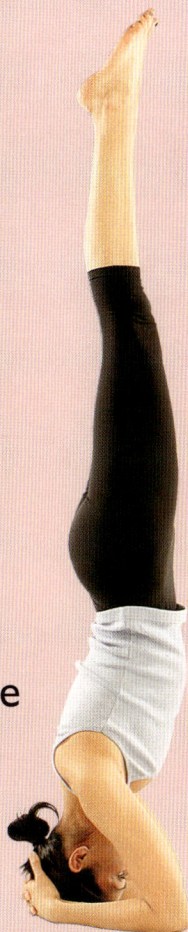

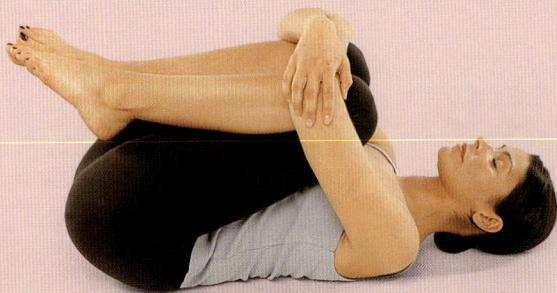

Child posture

For full instructions see pages 38–9.

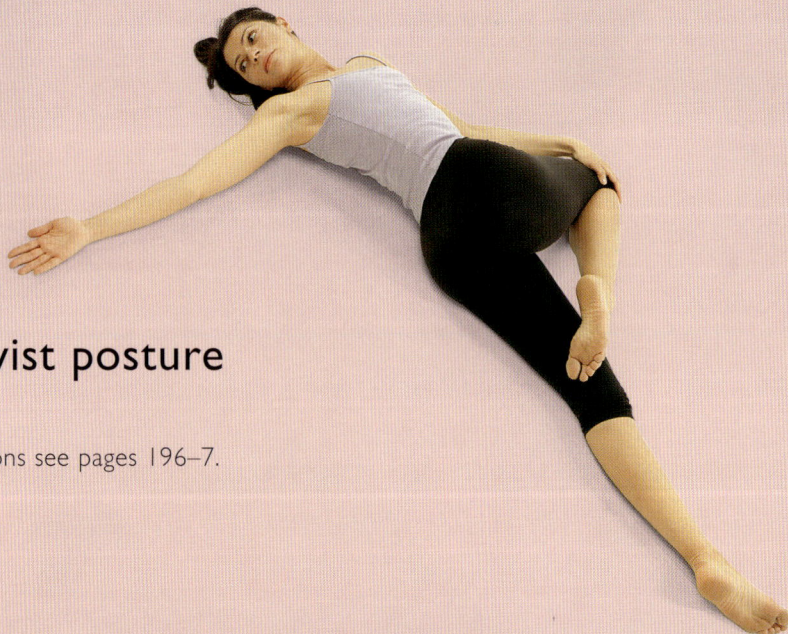

Supine twist posture

For full instructions see pages 196–7.

Half spinal twist posture

For full instructions see pages 194–5.

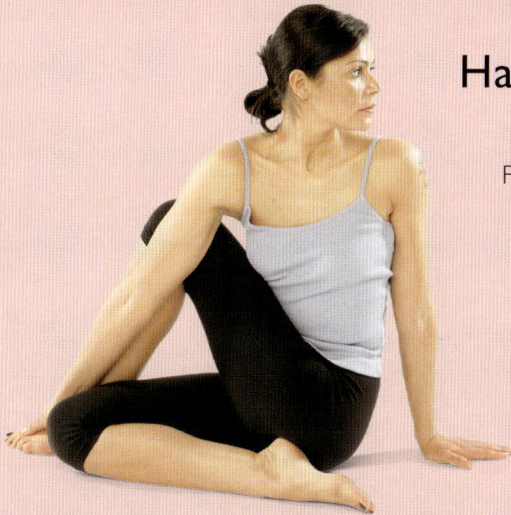

Half-lotus or
Lotus posture

Sit for 20 minutes using one of the meditation techniques from Chapter Eight. Switch legs if the posture becomes uncomfortable. For full instructions see pages 230–3.

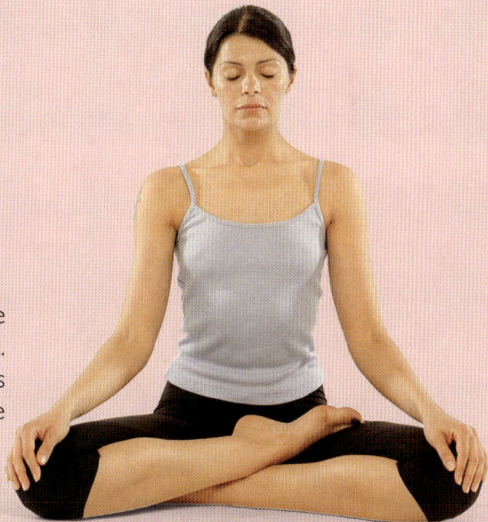

"Teachers open the door, but you must enter by yourself."

Chinese proverb

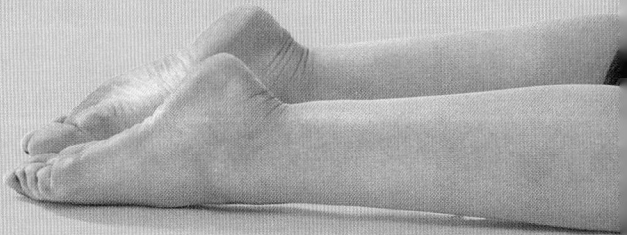

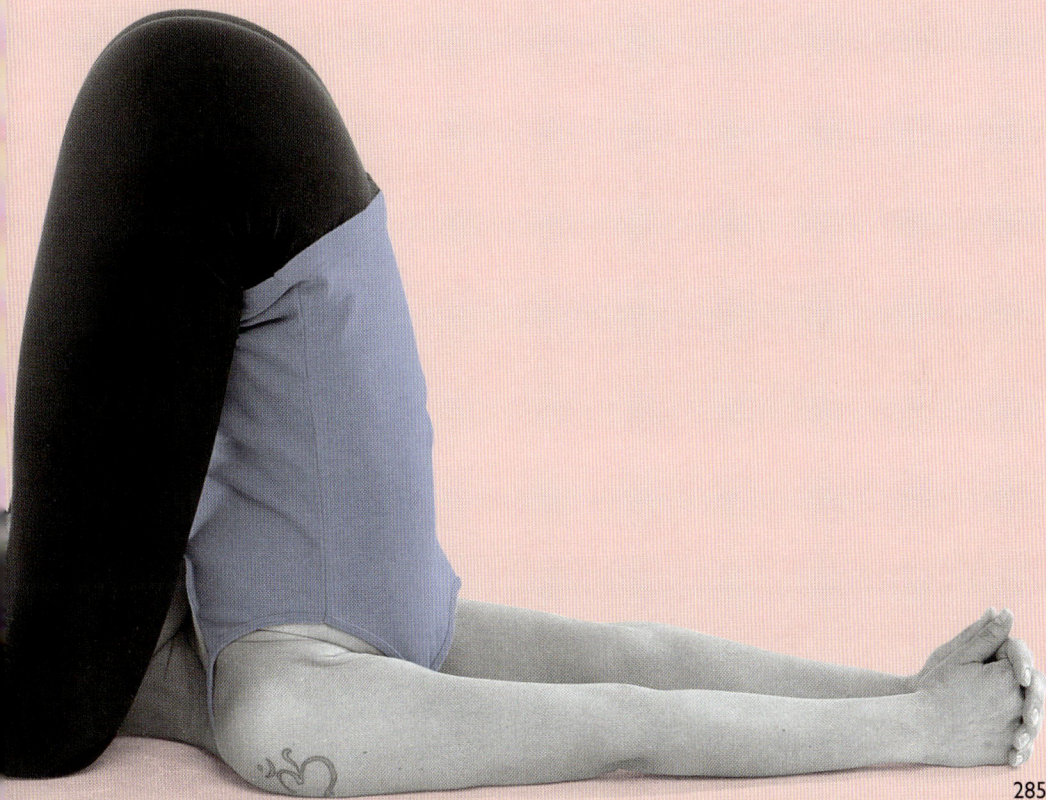

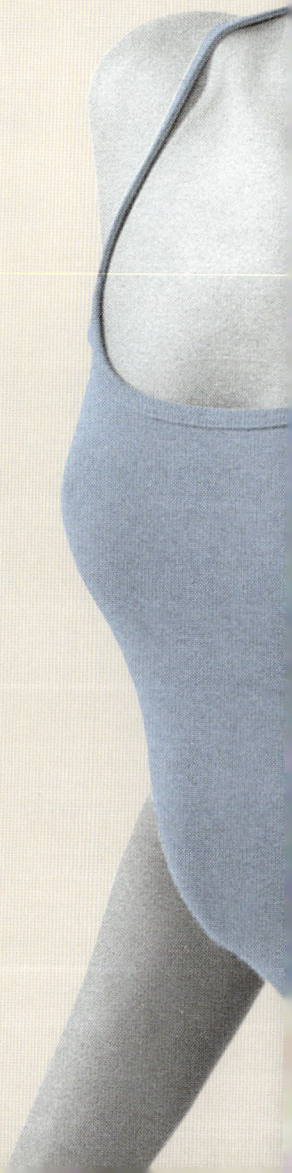

sun
salutations

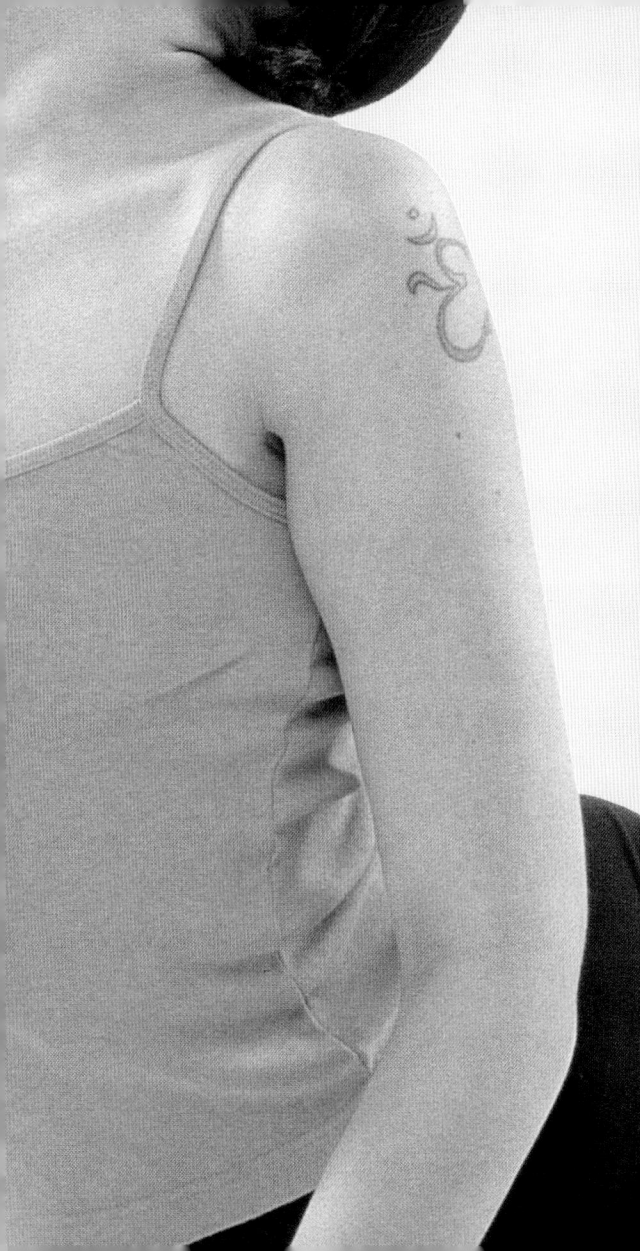

chapter 10

shivandana style

The Sun Salutation is a series of postures done in sequence. I have illustrated the Shivandana and Ashtanga styles (two versions). In both cases the Salutation is performed in time with the breath. You can use it as a morning energiser, or as a warm-up.

Stand in Tadasana with your heels and toes touching. Bring the hands together in prayer position.

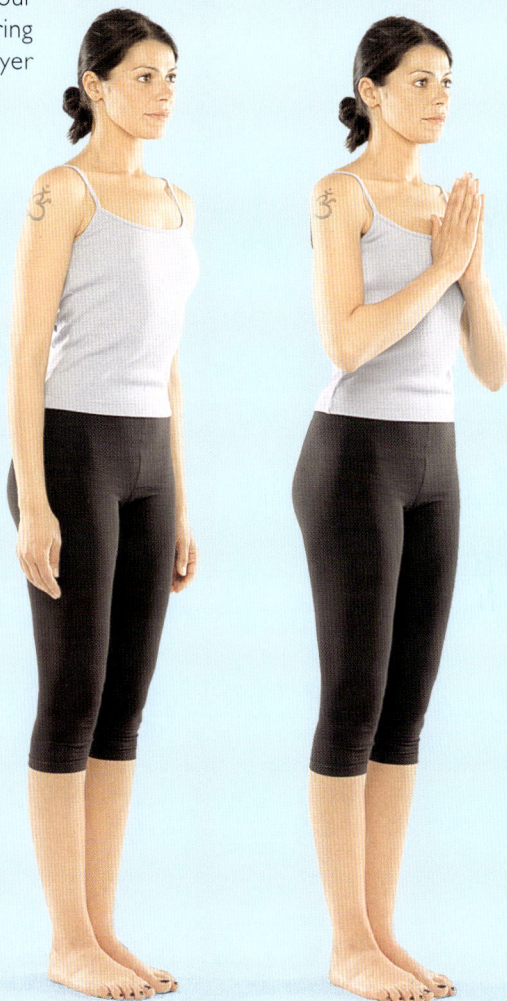

2 Breathe in and raise your arms up over your head, bending back as far as possible.

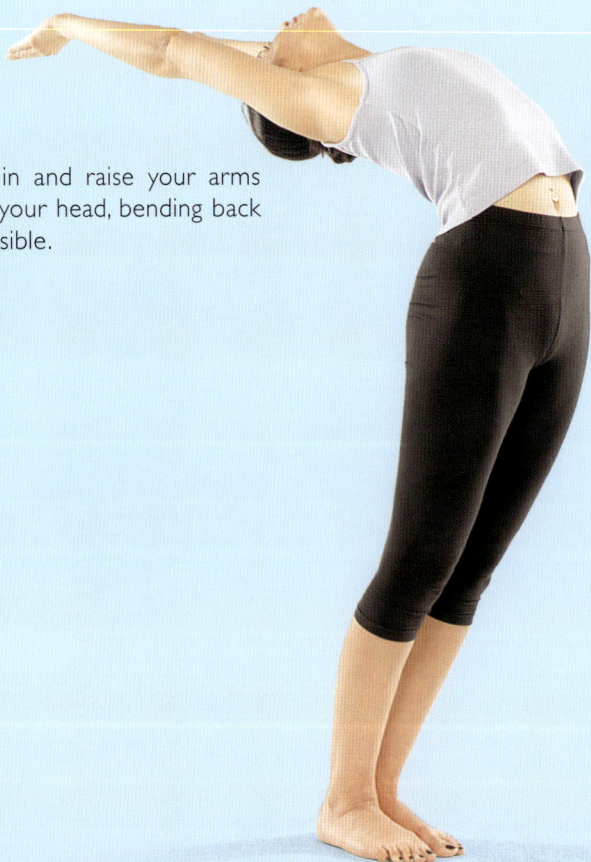

3 Breathe out, bend forward from the hips, and place your hands on the floor bringing your head to your knees. Beginners will have to bend their knees to achieve this position.

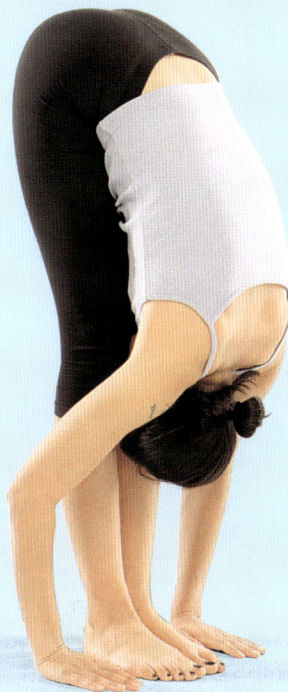

4 Breathe in and step back with your right leg, extending the toes of your right foot. Raise your head. Breathe out bring your left foot back next to your right. Your body is now in a press-up position. Place your knees, chest, and forehead on the floor.

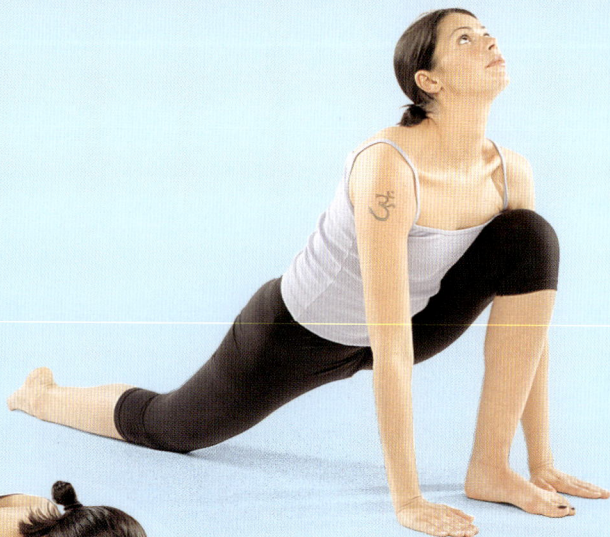

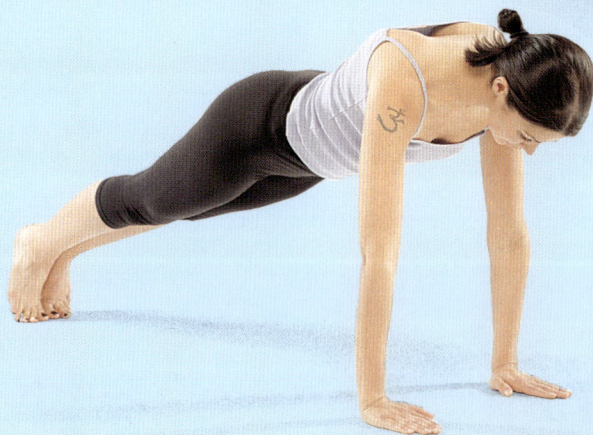

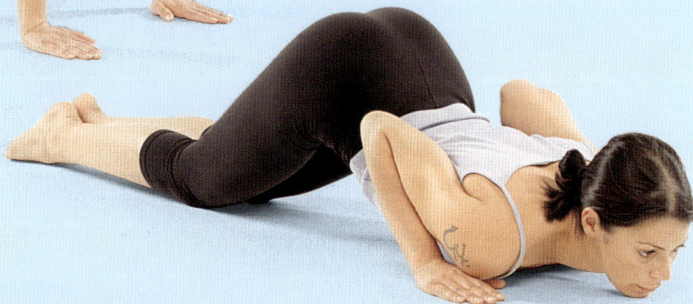

5 Breathe in as you slide forward into the Serpent pose (see pages 132–3), with your upper body raised off the floor on slightly bent arms. Tilt your head back if comfortable.

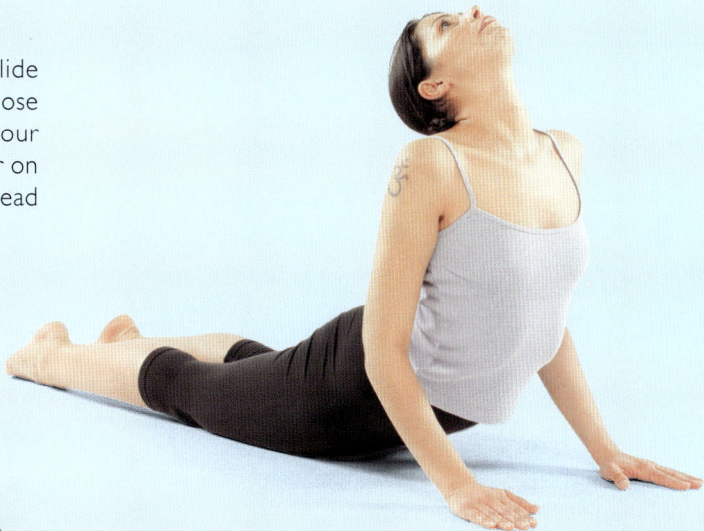

6 Breathe out, roll back onto your feet into an inverted V position (known as Downward dog pose).

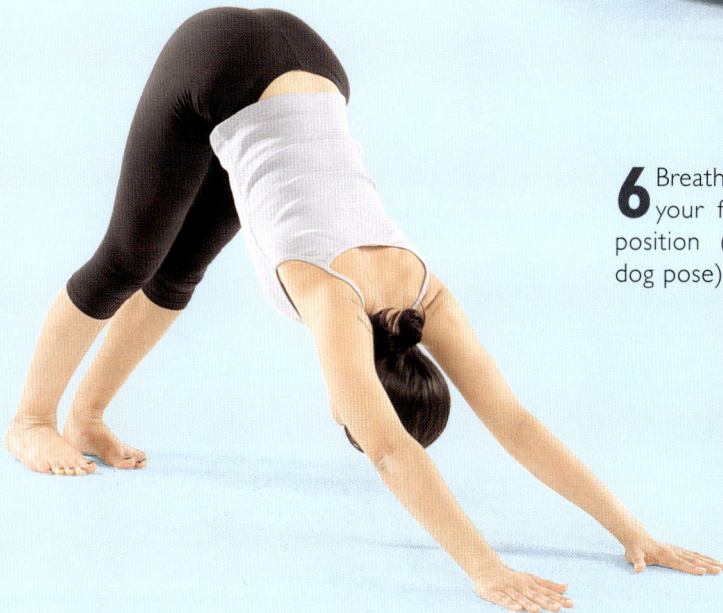

7 Breathe in and bend your right knee and step in between your hands. Breathe out and bring your left foot up to meet the right. Touch the head to the knees (with bent knees if necessary).

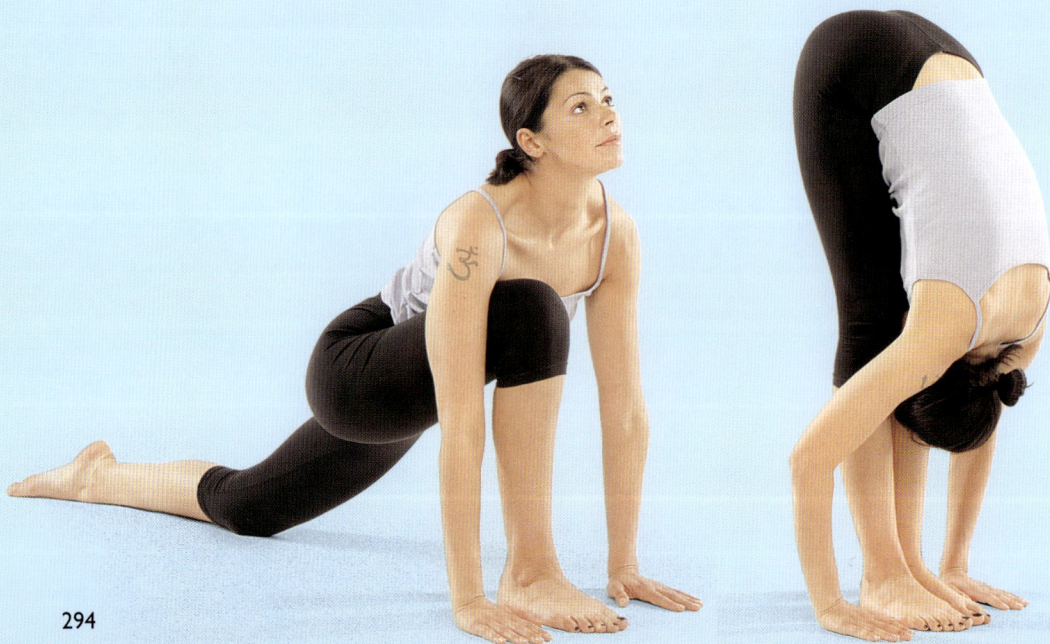

8 Breathe in, raise your arms and body into a backward bend. Breathe out and return to Tadasana. Repeat the whole cycle, leading with your left leg.

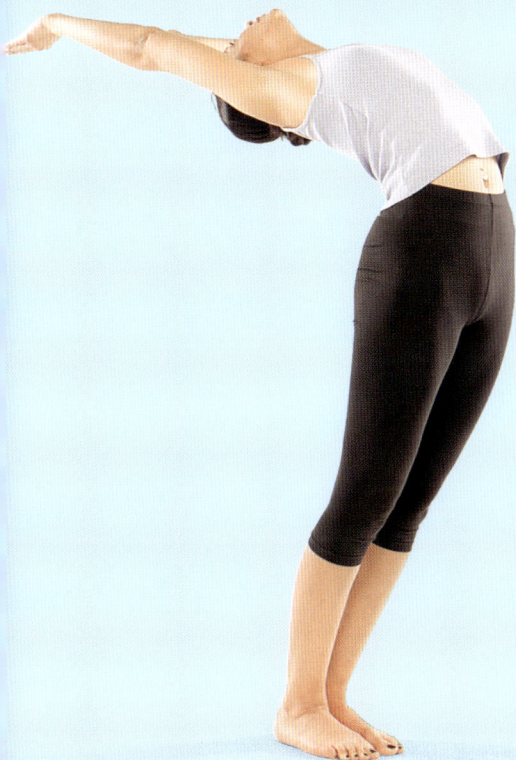

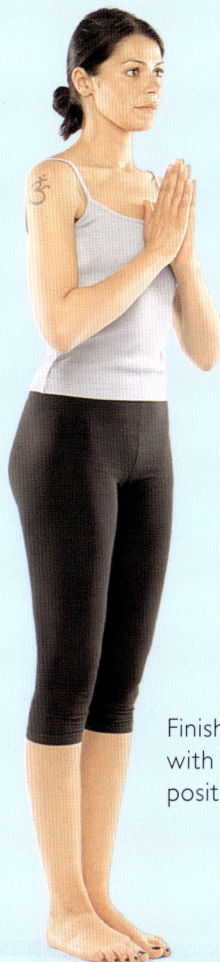

Finish by returning to Tadasana with your hands in prayer position.

295

"He who has faith, who is committed, and whose senses are under control, gains knowledge, and having obtained it, he quickly attains supreme peace."

Bhagavad Gita

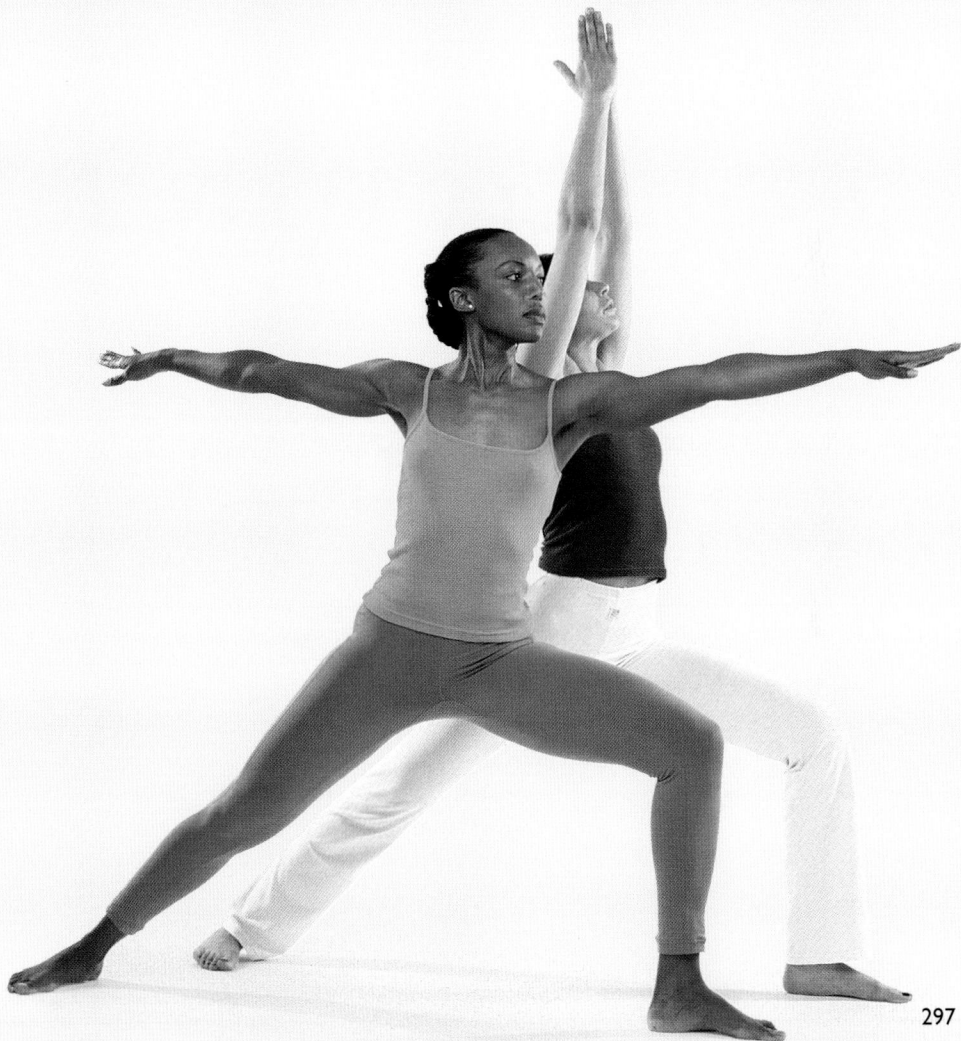

ashtanga style I

You will see many similarities with the Shivananda style salutation, but the performance of the movements is very different. Where the Shivananda is precise and slow, the Ashtanga salutation is powerful and dynamic. Use the Ujjayi breath (see page 67) when performing the Ashtanga Sun Salutation.

Stand in Tadasana with your heels and toes touching. Bring the hands together in the prayer position. Breathe in and raise your arms up over your head.

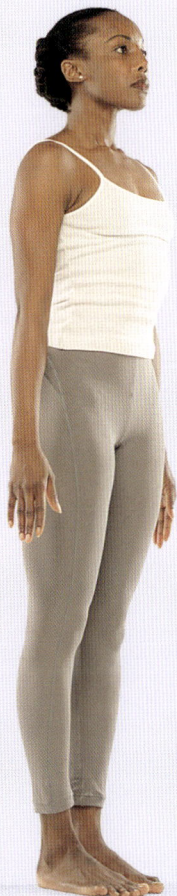

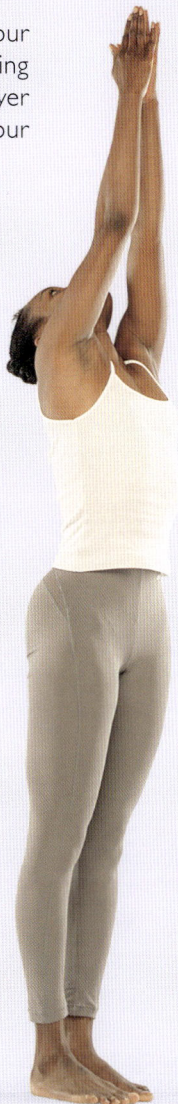

2 Breathe out, bend forward from the hips, and place your hands on the floor bringing your head to your knees. Beginners will have to bend their knees to achieve this position.

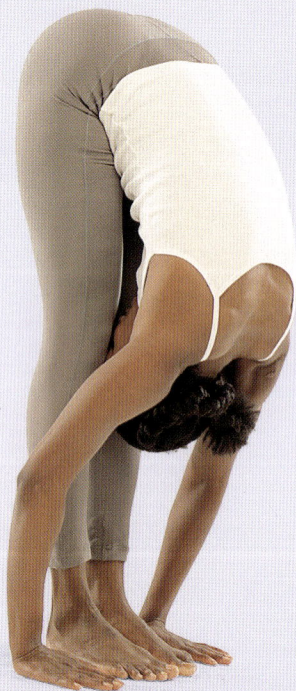

3 Breathe in, lift your head and look forward, trying to stretch and flatten your back. You hands are on their fingertips.

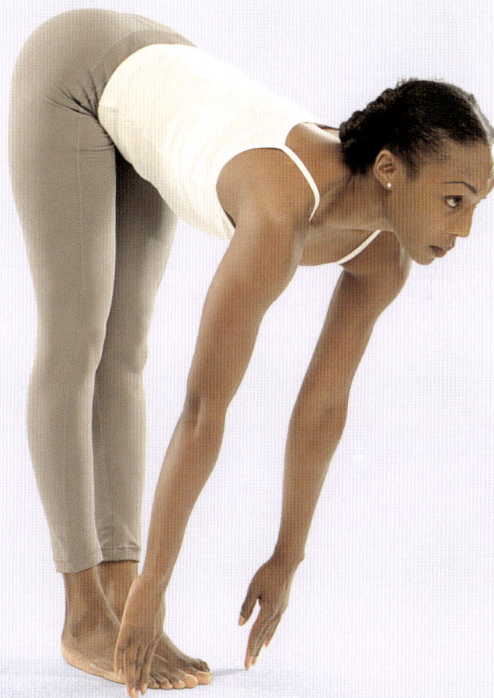

4 Breathe out, step or jump back so that your legs are straight behind you and your body is in a press-up position. Hold your breath as you lower your body a few inches from the floor.

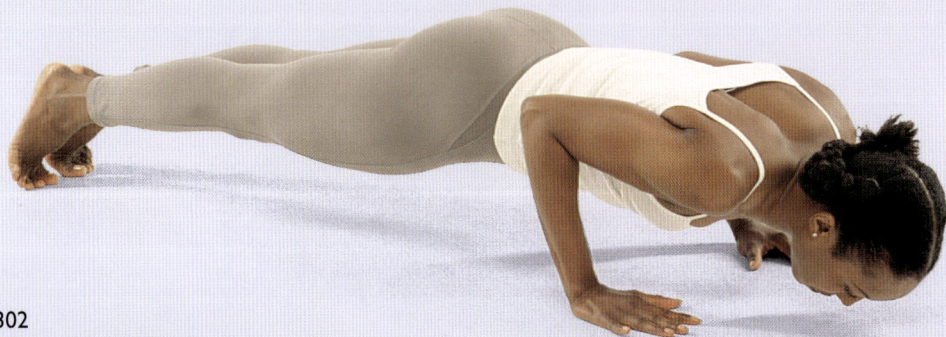

5 Breathe in as you slide through your hands into the Upward dog posture, which resembles the Serpent posture, but in which the legs and hips are held off the floor and the body is supported on the hands and the top of the extended feet.

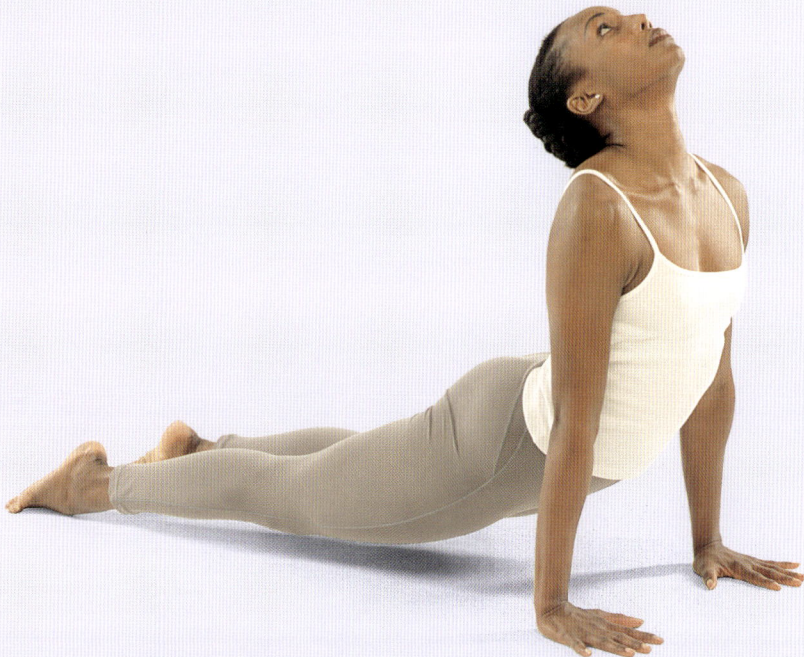

6 Breathe out as you move into the Downward dog posture, making your body into an inverted V, with both your hands and feet flat on the ground and, your back flat. Look through your legs or up at your navel.

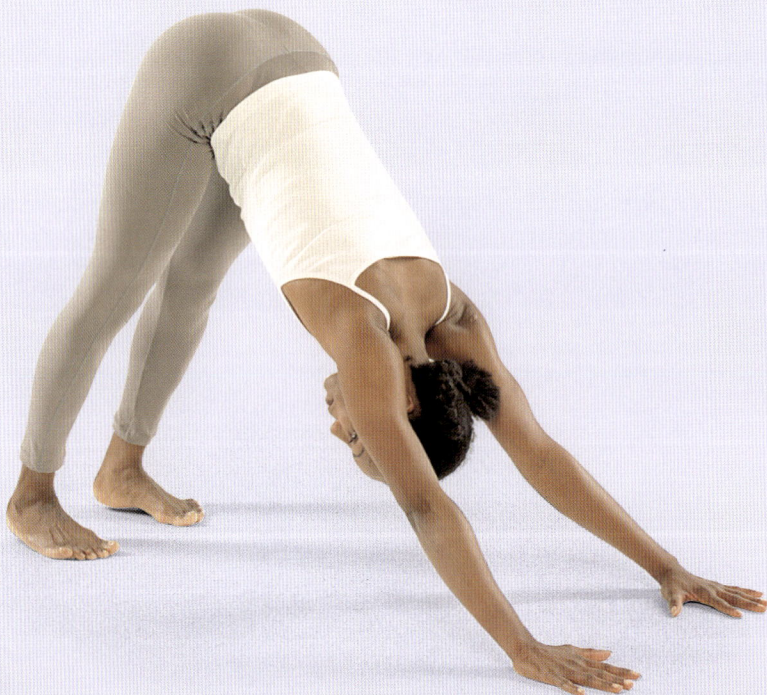

7 Breathe in, look up through your arms and step or jump forward so that your feet are between your hands with your head on your knees. Breathe out.

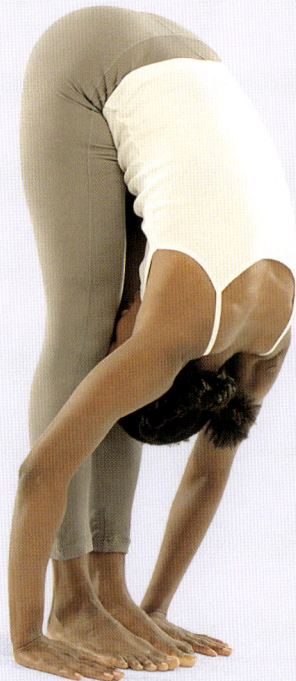

8 Breathe in as you look forward. Stretch and flatten your back. Breathe out, lower your head to your knees.

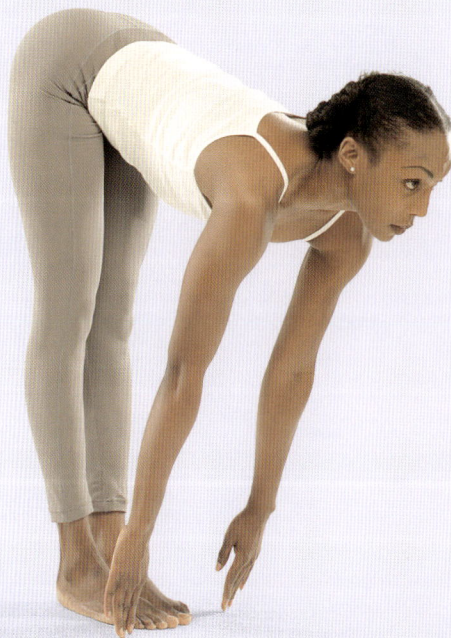

9 Breathe in as you stretch upward, bringing your arms together over your head.

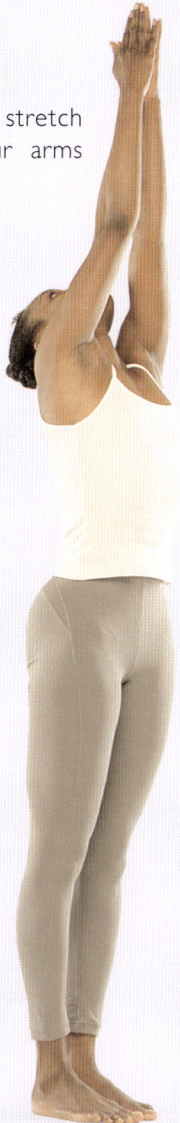

10 Breathe out, lower your hands to prayer position. Finish in Tadasana in preparation for the next Sun Salutation.

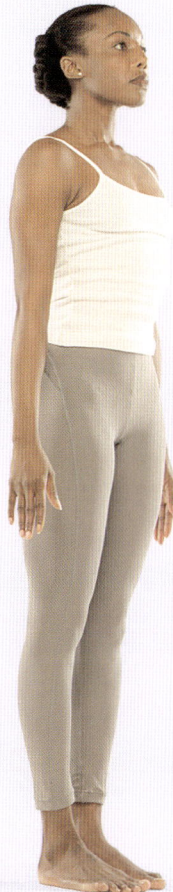

ashtanga style II

This Ashtanga variation of the Sun Salutation includes Virabhadrasana I, the Warrior posture (see pages 84–5) and a variation in the standing position at the beginning (see second picture opposite). Use the Ujjayi breath as in the Ashtanga I Sun Salutation.

1 Stand in Tadasana with your heels and toes touching. Breathe out as you bring your hands in prayer position. Breathe in, bend your knees as shown, and raise your arms up over your head, palms touching.

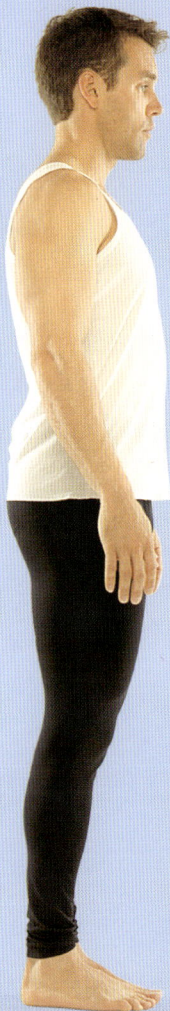

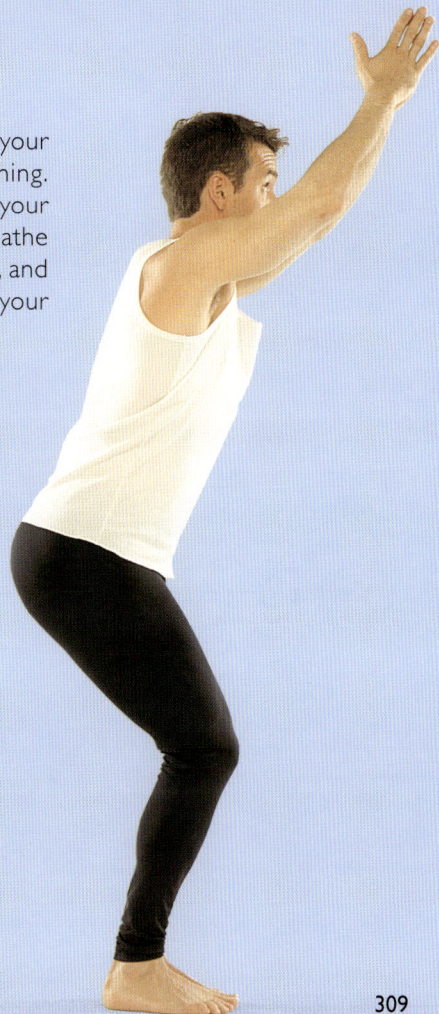

2 Breathe out, bend forward from the hips, and place your hands on the floor bringing your head to your knees. Beginners will have to bend their knees to achieve this position.

3 Breathe in, lift your head and look forward, trying to stretch and flatten your back. Your hands are on their fingertips.

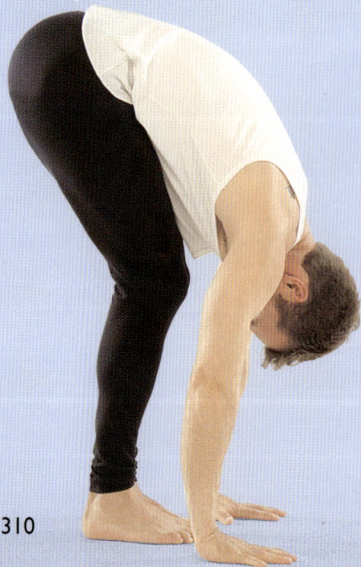

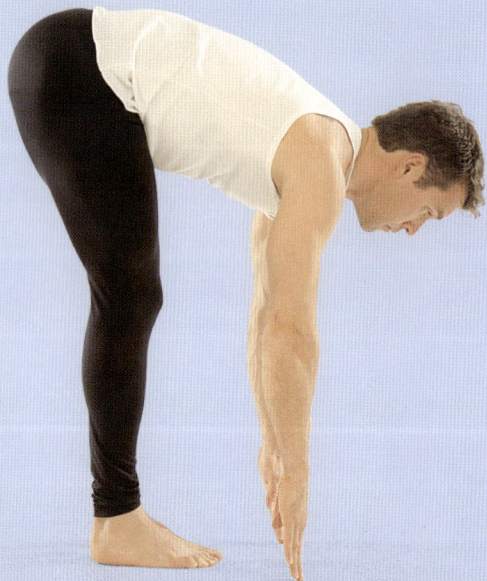

4 Breathe out, lower your head to your knees, jump or step back so that both feet are straight behind you and your body is in a press-up position. Hold your breath as you lower your body a few inches from the floor.

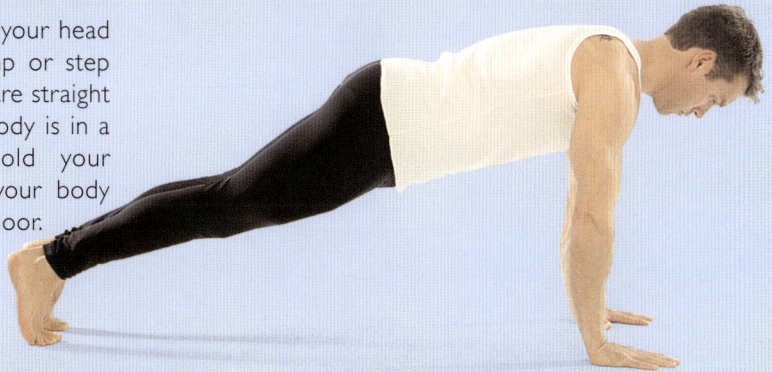

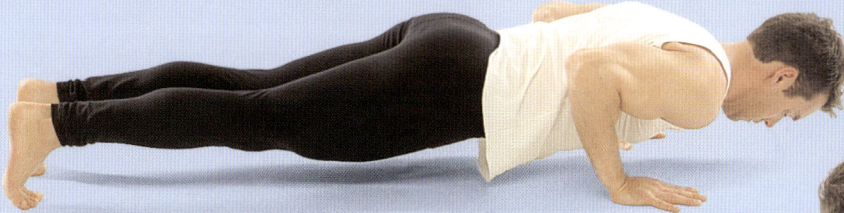

5 Breathe in as you slide forward into the Upward dog posture with your hips and legs raised off the floor, head titled back if you find it comfortable.

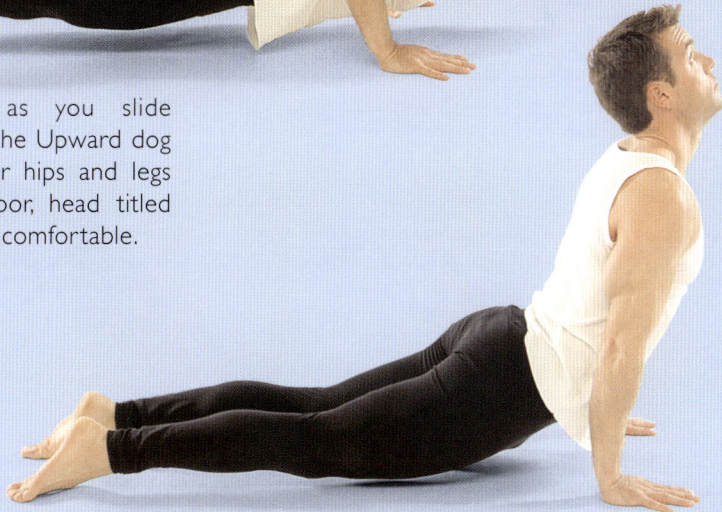

311

6 Breathe out, roll back onto your feet into an inverted V position (Downward dog posture).

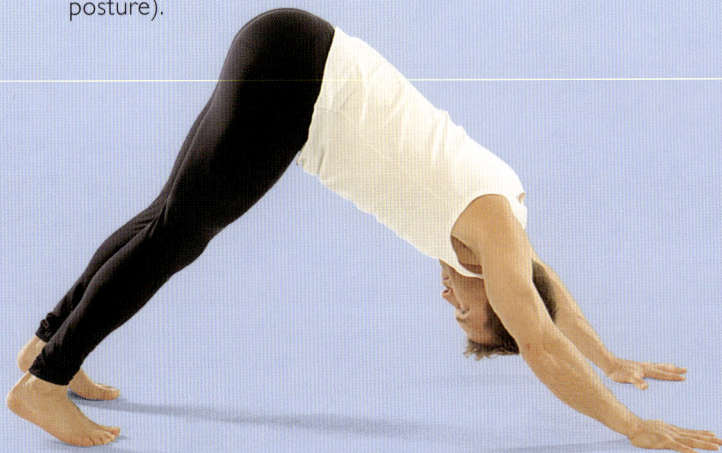

7 Breathe in, look up and step your right leg between your hands. Turn out your back foot, keeping it in line with your front foot. Raise your arms over your head into Warrior I posture (see pages 84–5).

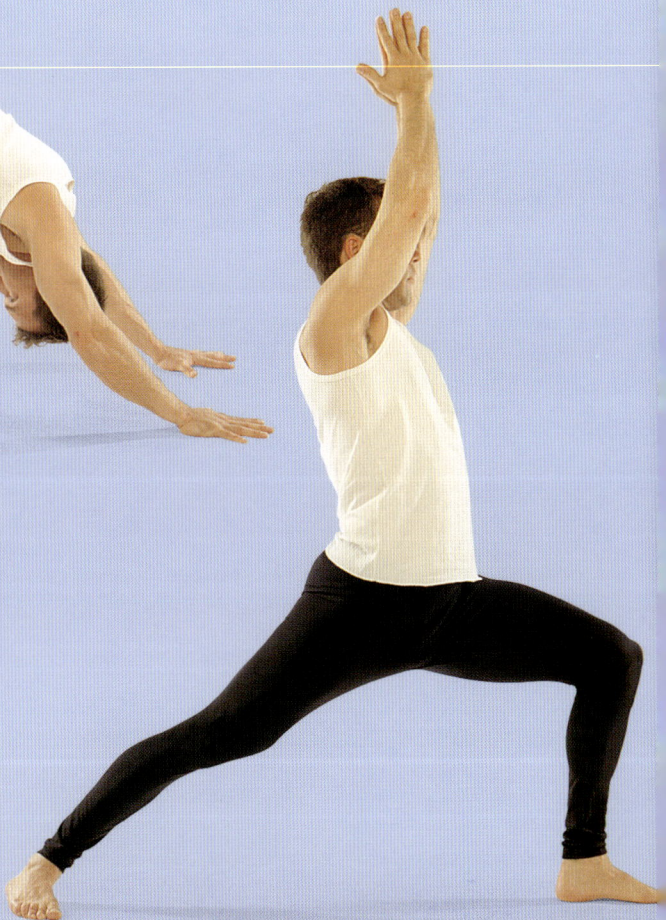

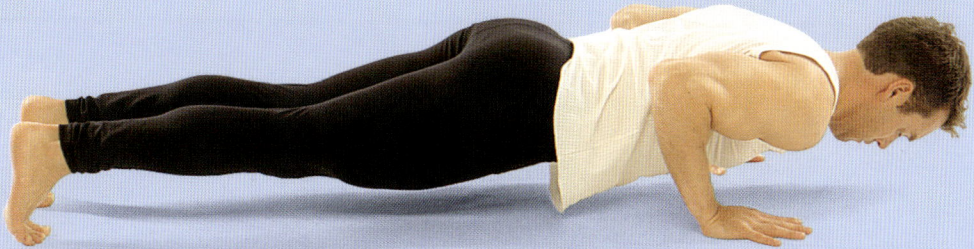

8 Breathe out. Place your hands on the ground on either side of your right foot. Place your right foot back next to the left so that you are in a press-up position.

9 Still breathing out, lower your body so that it is just off the ground. Breathe in as you slide through your hands into the Upward dog posture.

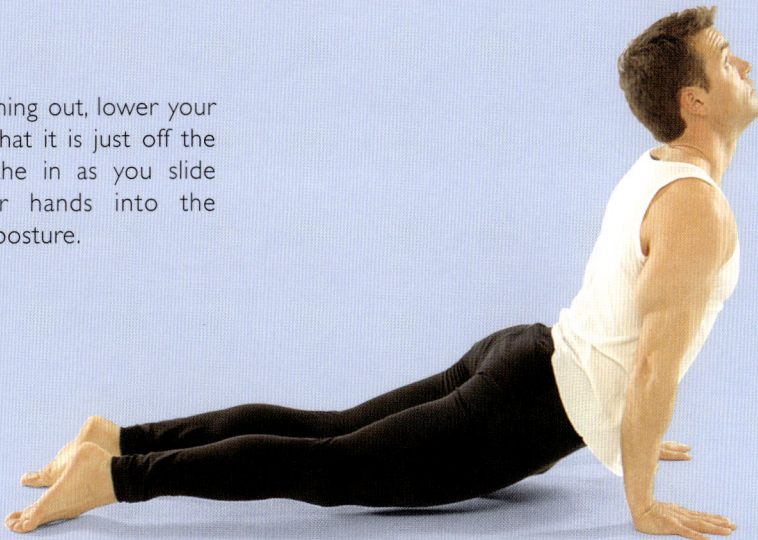

313

10 Breathe out, roll back onto your feet into an inverted V position (Downward dog posture).

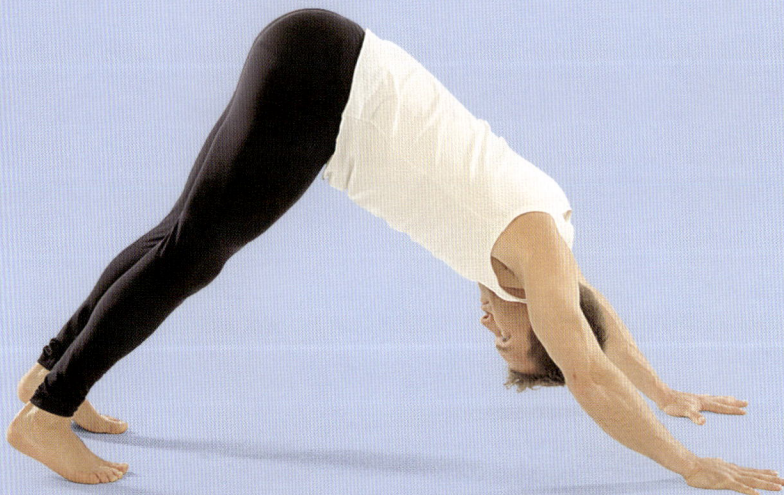

11 Breathe in, look through your hands and jump or step forward so that you are standing with your hands on the floor, trying to touch your knees with your head.

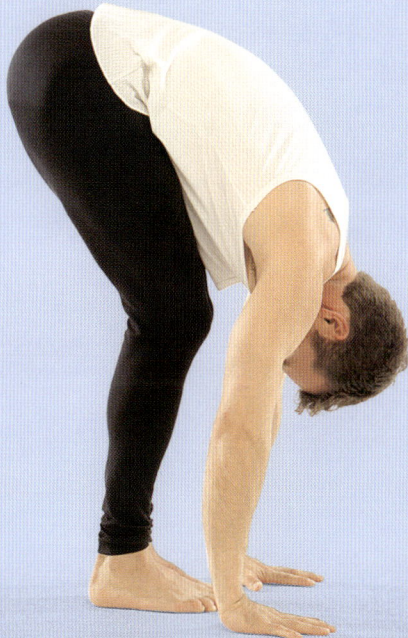

12 Breathe in, look up, stretch and flatten your back. Breathe out and lower your head to your knees (see overleaf).

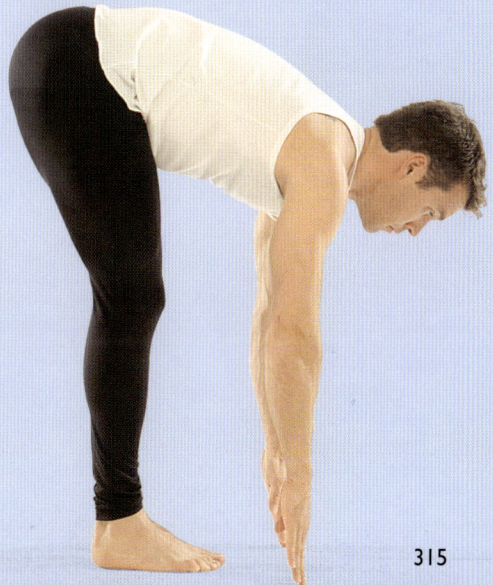

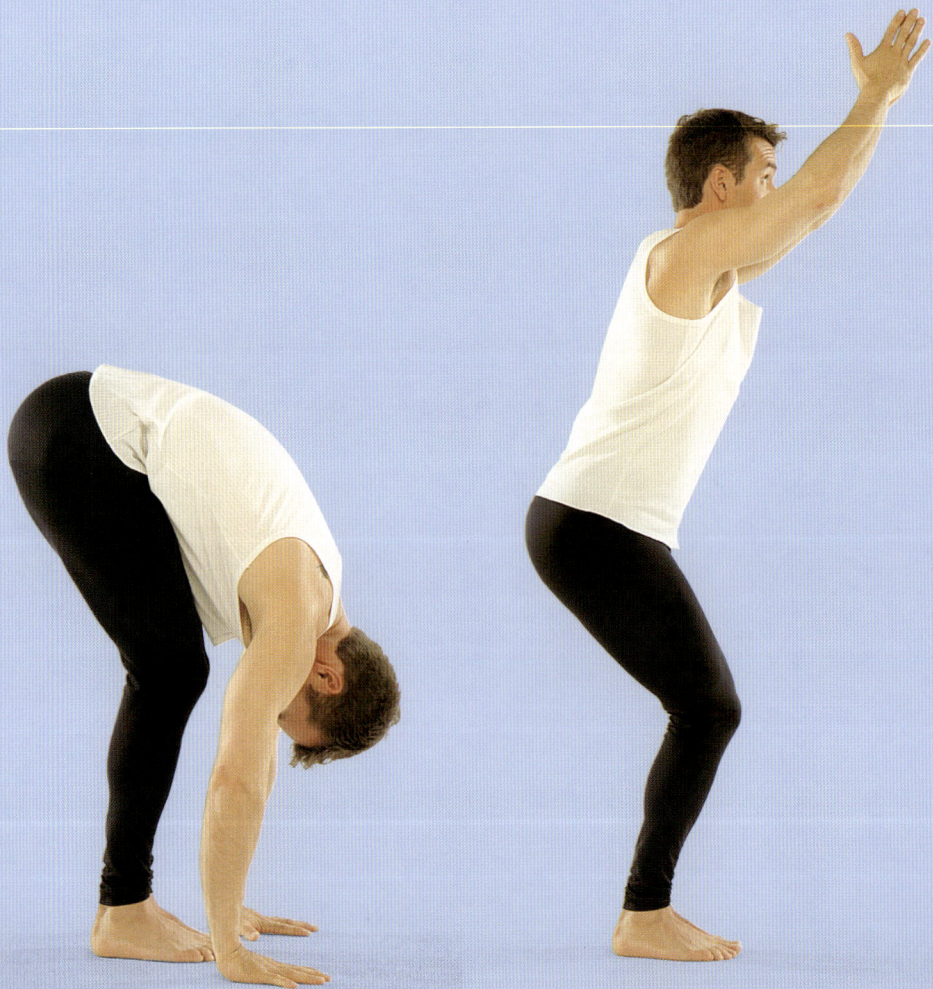

13 Breathe in, bend your knees as you raise your hands above your head, palms touching. Breathe out straightening your legs and lowering your hands into prayer position. Return to Tadasana in preparation for the next Sun Salutation, adding a Warrior I posture leading with the left leg as shown in the sequence.

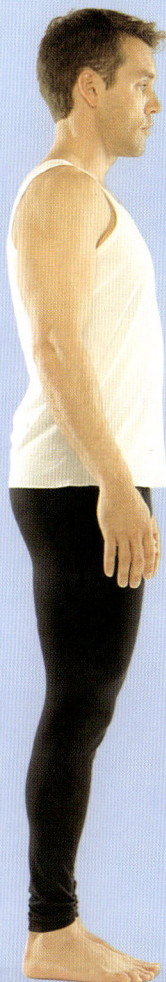

index